SONGS FOR THE FORGOTTEN

a psychiatrist's record

PRAISE FOR
Songs for the Forgotten

"Julia W. Burns manages to combine engagement with the trauma and clarity of issue and longed-for response for the healing and help of others. She echoes Dietrich Bonhoeffer, who once wrote that 'we need to listen with the ears of Christ to gain the right to speak the word of God.'"

—Rev. Russ Parker,
Director of 2Restore

"*Songs for the Forgotten* is a wake-up call to the world about the problem no one wants to talk about—the abuse of children. The purpose of this book is to shock our culture with the truth. To shock people into understanding not only how prevalent child abuse is, but how dangerous it is to pretend it's not happening. This book will open the eyes of the world to the dry rot that is destroying our children's safety."

—Will Burns,
CEO Ideasicle

"*Songs for the Forgotten* resonates, illuminates, and deeply moves us with its sharp particulars. Many of these wide-ranging narratives find you where you live. The stories read us as we read them; they locate the kind of experience we are responsive to, find certain areas of educated feeling, and touch upon our blind spots in a way that opens our eyes. There is redemptive love and a hope for healing."

—Peter Makuck,
Distinguished Professor Emeritus, East Carolina University

"Julia Burns shares her extensive experience with trauma in a way that helps the reader believe, make sense of, and engage with trauma stories they hear. By including her personal story, songwriting, and some of the traumatic stories she has heard, Burns creates readable flow that leaves room for rest and healing. Her book would be especially helpful for medical and therapeutic professionals, but is also accessible to laypersons who have encountered trauma either personally or among companions."

—Laura Dallas,
North Carolina Conference of the United Methodist Church

"A brave and empathetic journey into darkness, full of song and light."

—Robert Alden Rubin,
On the Beaten Path

"The natural revulsion that many of us feel when hearing these dark truths makes it too easy to turn away so that we don't have to face the brutality and brokenness of our own kind. If we don't believe, then we have no obligation to do anything, and as Dr. Burns makes crystal clear, the chain of suffering continues through the generations, a blight on so many lives and on our humanity."

—Leigh Anne Couch,
Former Managing Editor, Duke University Press

SONGS FOR THE FORGOTTEN

a psychiatrist's record

JULIA W. BURNS, MD

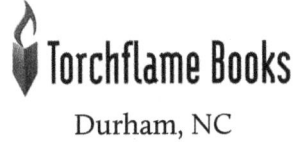

Torchflame Books
Durham, NC

Copyright © 2020 Julia W. Burns, MD
Songs for the Forgotten: a psychiatrist's record
Julia W. Burns, MD
www.juliaburns.org
jburns13@icloud.com

Published 2020, by Torchflame Books
    an Imprint of Light Messages Publishing
www.torchflame.com
Durham, NC 27713 USA
SAN: 920-9298
Paperback ISBN: 978-1-61153-371-2
E-book ISBN: 978-1-61153-372-9
Library of Congress Control Number: 2020906586

ALL RIGHTS RESERVED

No part of this publication may be reproduced, stored in a retrieval system, or transmitted in any form or by any means, electronic, mechanical, photocopying, recording, scanning, or otherwise, except as permitted under Section 107 or 108 of the 1976 International Copyright Act, without the prior written permission except in brief quotations embodied in critical articles and reviews.

Scripture quotations, unless otherwise indicated, are taken from THE MESSAGE, copyright © 1993, 2002, 2018 by Eugene H. Peterson. Used by permission of NavPress. All rights reserved. Represented by Tyndale House Publishers, Inc.

The Holy Bible, New International Version® (NIV®) Copyright © by Biblica, Inc.™

Names and personal details have been changed to protect the identities of people involved.

I dedicate these pages to Etta, Gerry, Henry, Mary Ellen, and to all who have been tormented before and since. This book is also dedicated to the abusers themselves, for I have learned that many perpetrators were victims first. And we cannot separate our healing prayers and love from one without hurting the other.

Storytelling

*I have heard it said
that when a woman
tells a story,*

*she becomes
both mother and child,
teller and listener,
curator and ticket holder,
to this event
that catalogues*

her life and destiny.

—Julia W. Burns, MD

FOREWORD

*The man who cries out against evil men
but does not pray for them
will never know the grace of God.*
—Saint Silouan the Athonite

IN 1874, NINE-YEAR-OLD MARY ELLEN WILSON was living in Hell's Kitchen, the underbelly of New York City, where she was beaten, neglected, and frequently chained to her bed. A religious missionary, Etta Wheeler, learned about Mary Ellen and attempted to rescue her. Police refused to investigate, and Child Charities were consulted, but they felt they lacked authority to interfere. No Child Protective Services existed, and there was no juvenile court.

Etta sought the advice of Henry Bergh, the founder of the American Society for the Prevention of Cruelty to Animals. Bergh asked his lawyer, Elbridge Gerry, to find a legal way to rescue the child. The lawyer used a law protecting animals to remove her from the guardians: they had Mary Ellen declared an "animal."

Following the successful rescue of Mary Ellen Wilson, Henry Bergh and Elbridge Gerry created a private charitable society devoted to child protection. The New York Society for the Prevention of Cruelty to Children became the world's first organization devoted exclusively to child protection.[1]

But change in the welfare of children was slow, and one hundred years later, in 1974, the *Comprehensive Textbook of Psychiatry* stated: "Incest is extremely rare, and does not occur in more than 1 in 1.1 million people." The editors went on to say that an incestuous relationship actually provided the victim a type of resilience in its aftermath: "Such incestuous activity diminishes the subject's chance of psychosis and allows for a better adjustment to the external world."[2]

In 1992, children could be diagnosed with anxiety or depression, but trauma was not believed to be a contributor to a child's function. "People didn't think babies could experience pain, and so doctors used to operate on them without anesthetic, and experts didn't think children could suffer from grief or depression," Dr. Nick Midgley said, in his book *Reading Anna Freud*.[3] Children's ability to suffer was a concept which developed slowly in the medical profession.

Extinguishing negative behaviors was the primary goal of therapy, not understanding life stories that created and sustained these behaviors. Often, the trauma history was dismissed or rarely incorporated into team meetings or evaluations, despite the fact that abuse in child welfare agencies was high.

My hope is that this book, these stories, these lives will put an end to the myth that child abuse is rare. Your reading of this book will help enhance understanding that if abuse is left unrecognized and untreated, it will continue to weave into the fabric of our culture and every individual, suffering will not end, and healing will be out of reach for both the abused and their abuser.

*You did it: you changed wild lament
into whirling dance;
You ripped off my black mourning band
and decked me with wildflowers.
I'm about to burst with song;
I can't keep quiet about you.
God, my God,
I can't thank you enough.*

—Psalm 30:11-12

INTRODUCTION

> *"My argument against God was that the universe
> seemed so cruel and unjust.
> But how had I got this idea of just and unjust?
> A man does not call a line crooked
> unless he has some idea of a straight line.
> What was I comparing this universe with
> when I called it unjust?"*
>
> —C.S. Lewis,
> *Mere Christianity*

I SING A SONG FOR THE ABUSED CHILD, the song no one wants to hear. I sing a song learned from a lifetime of listening as a child psychiatrist and as a patient in therapy—discerning fact from fiction, thoughts from emotions. I hope you will listen and learn, for it's the song of a child left alone. Who will feed her? Who will care? I know that song, and it is a song I'll gladly sing for the child who will never learn to trust, the child who suffered so much before birth that when she was born into her life of abuse, she had little chance. It's the song of so many who never had a childhood. It's also my song and my story—the story of someone who happened into a career at a child treatment facility, a career she never envisioned, one that threatened to sweep her away with the intensity of feelings that comes from healing traumatized patients. But wait, I'm starting at the end.

First, the story of my work at White Pines.

New Hampshire had a three-hundred-child welfare agency, White Pines, where I treated children and adolescents between the ages of six and eighteen who needed placement away from their families. All were in residential care because of aggression, running away, truancy, or sexual acting out. Our mission was to treat their out-of-control behaviors, allowing them to return to home and public school. As staff psychiatrist, my job included completing initial psychiatric evaluations, attending monthly treatment-team meetings, prescribing medications, overseeing nursing and social work staff, tracking lab data such as liver functions, creatinine, and blood counts, and monitoring children in foster homes. I was on-call twenty-four hours a day, seven days a week—for years. As the work demanded constant attention, so did the children and their stories.

If the extent of the invisible problem of childhood trauma is hard for you to believe, then you may have had a rare and safe childhood. Unfortunately, many have not. Perhaps you are one of these: one whose song will be sung in this book. It is my patient's stories that I want to share with *both* of you—the ones who might take a nurturing home for granted, and the ones who can't imagine what that home looks like.

I hope these stories teach people the truth about abuse without causing more pain. Some of you won't believe me, or will be shocked that the system could ignore or even perpetuate child maltreatment. Perhaps others have a story that makes believing mine far too easy. As I tell my story and sing these songs, I will carry you into the world of trauma so that you may understand how much healing is required and how loving attention from adults can protect children.

As academic institutions graduate doctors with little sensitivity toward trauma, abuse will continue to thrive. The medical world in the late 1980s and early 1990s was in such denial about the reality of physical and sexual abuse that the impact of childhood trauma on behavior and mental health was not considered. Even today, psychiatrists in training often skip the study of trauma, spending weeks on schizophrenia instead.

According to the U.S. Department of Health and Human Services, childhood sexual abuse affects one in four girls and one in six boys. Schizophrenia occurs in less than 1 percent of the normal population, but studying biological illnesses you can medicate is more appealing than studying abuse. My own work with patients leads me to suspect that this number is actually much higher, especially for boys, as they frequently forget or minimize their abuse.

Consider this healthcare crisis in the context of a medical system that reimburses for cardiac bypass surgery, but shows less interest in preventing heart disease through nutrition or exercise; or one that graduates pediatric residents who spend hours in the neonatal intensive care unit placing arterial lines—a skill they will probably not need in a busy pediatric private practice—but never sends them to a lecture on bed wetting or thumb sucking, which they will treat daily. This makes our current disregard for physical and sexual abuse more understandable—and more fixable.

Working at White Pines as medical director brought this crisis of faith front and center as I listened to children describe being molested, and read reports of young children who were groomed for sex from birth. I could no longer deny my impotence nor condone what I understood as God's neglect.

Despite walking with my family every Sunday to church, I struggled to *love* the God I worshipped. Consumed with anger, I felt a rising despair: my spirit was dying. Often, I fell to my knees, begging Christ to make it different, to change human behavior so children could be safe. But I only heard silence.

As indignant as I was about the number of children I was caring for who were mistreated, I was increasingly bewildered about the staff's lack of understanding about how trauma affects behavior. Many times, children were reacting to requests from teachers and staff with rage and opposition because they were afraid. Their fear stemmed from childhood abuse, yet few staff workers made this connection even as behaviors escalated: throwing chairs or books in the classroom, destroying bedrooms, or hitting a friend or teacher.

Residents or children who lived in on-grounds cottages, and foster children, who received therapy and medication management with the agency but lived off campus with families, could not gain privileges with these behaviors. They were restricted in school and not allowed freedom for after-school activities. These restrictions made them more aggressive. All the while, neurological damage from trauma controlled their every action, and yet this was not acknowledged.

My nights were filled with the echoes of a child's voice crying, "I didn't mean to be a bad girl. It's hard to stand in the corner for hours." My sleep was splintered with images of Bill, the latest admission to White Pines, and his burned back. It had been scalded by his mother because he had forgotten to do the dishes.

My instinct was to flee White Pines and stop listening to the stories that were hurting and overwhelming me. I was not aware of the now well-documented phenomenon of *vicarious,* or *secondary,* trauma, which is considered an epidemic among therapists. It occurs when the person treating the patient becomes injured by the experience of listening and helping, effectively sustaining post-traumatic stress disorder (PTSD). I was suffering from a malady that, at the time, had no name. I was afraid to quit my work, yet fearful of remaining: Paralyzed. I knew that the listening had wounded me, that my anger and outrage was destructive, but I had no idea what was wrong or how to fix it.

Sensitivity and intuition were my gift and my curse. Able to receive many stories with belief, from a young age, I listened with earnestness and compassion.

As an adult, my patients' traumas poured out: beatings and neglect, days without food or supervision, children looking for parents who never came home, or came home late, drunk, and unable to provide nourishment or love; stories of favorite priests, uncles, or teachers who insinuated themselves into the family, only to grope and ultimately penetrate the children or force oral sex upon them. My patients had split themselves into many different people in order to block such memories. When we met, they began to surrender their stories to someone who believed, in hopes that they could reintegrate and one day become whole.

One day, I knew it was over; the day I could not see a way out came. You've heard of the dark night of the soul. Well, this was my midnight, and I was gasping for breath.

Although I stayed in school until my mid-thirties, studying human behavior, I found myself poorly equipped for the thousands of stories that children of all ages told me of neglect and abuse—emotional, physical, and sexual. If my patient's couldn't tell me with words, their bodies couldn't lie. Their rage, aggression, mood swings, dissociation, hyperactivity, learning disabilities, and eating disorders spoke loudly.

But the story that led to my resignation, the song that a mother sang of a night with her baby, Ginny, went like this:

Her eyes were downcast.
She was weary, wearing unwashed rags,
sullen and dull
as she recounted the echo of a story
she didn't want to repeat,
didn't want to believe—like the judge
who said it hadn't happened.

She gasped for the breath to tell the story
of that night, and the story
of what was to follow.

Awakening to her baby's choking,
she turned on the light,
exposing the child's father,
his face contorted, penis engorged.

Her baby, in rooting for a mother's breast,
had found a monster.

*No one believed her,
and I've wanted to forget this
—both the crying and the choking,
the story and the disbelieving—many times.*

The mother had the courage to tell this truth to her case worker. Her case worker reported the incident to legal aid, and the father was charged with child sexual abuse. The disbelief came from the judge, and the case was thrown out of court because he didn't think it was possible. This book stands as evidence that it is. Your reading and believing brings justice to Ginny and her mother, denying the judge his not guilty verdict, denying the lie that infants cannot be abused just because they cannot speak and testify.

Continuing this work long after I should have stopped, I believed erroneously that if I didn't listen, no one would. And thus, I became a healer who needed healing. Loving my work and my patients, I persevered even as doubts arose regarding the magnitude of the problem and the limited effectiveness of my medical education and the child welfare system. My fury mounted, and I challenged a God who would create a world filled with traumatized children and a treatment system that couldn't heal them and didn't seem to care. "God, anyone could have done better," I prayed.

After a decade of listening, I was wounded, too. Once I experienced how massive the problem was, it was crushing not to be able to do more to eradicate it. I've spent much time in prayer and repentance, because even though I know it's not my fault, it feels like it should be someone's failing, and surely someone's responsibility.

Symptoms that I diagnosed in patients emerged to a lesser degree in me—anger, edginess, withdrawal, numbness, and isolation—but I had no doctor treating my trauma. My supervisor and I met weekly to review difficult cases, but we never spoke of secondary trauma. Neither of us knew of that syndrome. PTSD was primarily a disorder for war veterans—what once had been called *shell shock*. Shell shock in a child seemed far-fetched. At the time, the Diagnostic and Statistical Manual of Mental Disorders (DSM) did not even include a category for chronic trauma in children, much less in therapists. Now the manual that psychiatrists use includes categories for acute and chronic PTSD, and today there is a burgeoning interest in the epidemic of secondary trauma in therapists, with much new research on the horizon.

As the problems of working at a large welfare agency began creeping into my family life, I recognized the need to resign. My patients, acutely sensitive to abandonment, knew I was suffering and that I might leave them. On rounds in the morning, my patients asked if I felt safe, and I said yes. But the answer was no. I wasn't safe, and neither was Ginny when the judge allowed her father to return home.

Six years after the judge said not guilty, she was admitted to the residential treatment facility at White Pines. Ginny and I met frequently in the padded time-out room. Her rage was packed into a flashback so violent that the biting, spitting, and pissing told the story without words. And now she was in my time-out room, stripping and urinating on my childcare workers, trying to wash herself clean, because no one heard. Listen so you can hear her and believe the unarticulated story in these choking sounds. Not even Lithium, Haldol, and Ativan can suppress the sounds of choking now.

I sing this song because both she and her mother's voices have been robbed. That's why I am writing this book, telling you the stories they told me, verbally or nonverbally, so the lie of denial can die, so the wounded can rise above their stories. These songs of lamentation will release us, because before healing can occur, trauma requires remembering and recounting to someone who believes.

Join me in the listening, the believing, the mourning, and forgiveness, so that together we can create light in this darkness.

BIRTH

*It's a fact: darkness isn't dark to you;
night and day, darkness and light,
they're all the same to you.
Oh yes, you shaped me
first inside, and then out;
you formed me in my mother's womb.
I thank you, High God—you're breathtaking!*

—Psalm 139:12-13

BORN IN EASTERN NORTH CAROLINA, the third daughter, I grew up to be a healer and a physician, but not always both at the same time. There was a long tradition of faith healers in my family, and I followed in that practice. It was not unusual for someone to call my uncle during Sunday lunch, requesting that he stop their bleeding or remove a wart. Thus, my DNA led me to be a healer before becoming a doctor. Bandaging my dolls broken bones, conducting funerals for baby birds, and giving Momma a back rub were my initial forays into healing.

My formal scientific training led me to surrender almost all my healing power; the rigid method of medical school pushed aside my intuitive, artistic talents. For example, I did not play the piano or sing during medical training. Maybe there was no time. Or perhaps the rigors of forty-five-hour weeks in anatomy labs and lecture halls created a thinking brain which could not transform easily to the creative brain. Thankfully, I retained just enough intuitive sensitivity to claim it again, although it took years. As relationships grew between my patients and me, healing was created which combined science and art, and the return of those mysterious gifts allowed my destiny to be fulfilled.

Conjuring up moments of my own childhood and adolescence so you can understand the formation of a trauma healer seems fair: a reciprocation for the intimate sharing of our childhoods, both mine and my patients. However, I don't prefer talking about myself. The privacy necessary since hearing these stories and developing PTSD is complete and creates safety. I'd rather tell you about my patients than myself—the suffering and triumphs of the children, teenagers, and adults I've treated for the past thirty years.

But maybe you have ideas of how a child psychiatrist develops. Perhaps you're interested in glimpses into my childhood. So I'm opening the window for you, reluctantly but fully.

After seven days of bedrest in the hospital, Momma climbed into the cab of Daddy's pickup truck with me in her arms, and we traveled the short distance to our home in Sims, North Carolina. Penny, my almost two-year-old sister, sat in the middle, patting my head.

"It's okay, girl. You're going to be fine," she crooned, as I fretted.

Our home was situated on a crossroads—a farming town where Daddy sold insurance, and Momma ran the office of a seed farm company nearby. Momma loved to tell the story about how we couldn't nurse and how I couldn't hold down formula, either.

"We must have tried six or seven kinds of milk, and nothing agreed with you, Julia. Dr. Grant ordered soy milk to keep you from wasting completely away."

That first summer, Momma laid me out in the yard, on a bedspread, without a diaper because my skin was so "red and angry. You were so scrawny. Lord, how we prayed."

Momma believed infants should be baptized at six weeks of age, so around March 1957, we stood by the baptismal font of the Buckhorn United Methodist Church in Kenly, North Carolina, dedicating ourselves to Christ and renouncing evil. I must have been listening mightily when the minister asked if I accepted the freedom and power God gave me to resist evil, injustice, and oppression in whatever forms they presented themselves, because that vow created a backdrop for the life to come. Jesus, shepherding his flock, loomed over us from a stained glass window as I was marked as Christ's own and sealed as his forever. The congregation promised to uphold me. And together, with my family and godparents, we pronounced in unison that life should be lived in forgiveness and love. Lived out in a community of believers.

Penny was probably dressed in a yellow cotton dress that my Dad's sister, Aunt Deek, made, hair curled and white anklets turned down. I may have worn the lovely white christening gown that she and Hope, my oldest sister, had worn years prior.

Hope, born with a neural tube defect which caused hydrocephalus, died when she was one year old, never coming home.

Daddy held me, quieting any fussiness that may have rung out as the water ran from my forehead, into my eyes. I don't believe I cried, though. I imagine I was stricken by the Holy Spirit right there at the baptismal font, silenced and in awe—the first, but not the last time that would happen.

My deep brown, almost black eyes belonged to Daddy, my sassiness to Momma, and my strong will was attributable to both. Although I was much wanted, a boy would have been better. And that made me who I am. When the grass needed mowing or

Daddy rode out in the country, I got to go. No brothers blocked my journey into the world my father inhabited.

There was laughter in my family, but not a lot of nonsense. Both my parents were raised on tobacco farms and knew that before the harvest, you had to plant and sucker. Neither shirked hard labor, their years together yielding a plentiful bounty through constant work. My sister Penny and I are part of that abundance.

When I was two years old, Daddy was asked to manage the Farm Bureau Insurance agency in Robeson County. He knew it was the poorest county in North Carolina. Nicknamed the deadliest community in the state by the local newspaper. Drugs, poverty, gangs, and domestic violence were prevalent. One-third black, one-third Lumbee Indian, and one-third white, diversity was a way of life, not a notion. Education was ranked last in the state. Tobacco and textiles provided most folks' living, and those industries were gone by the time I graduated from high school.

But Daddy wanted a chance for something bigger. Wanted to dust the dirt off his farming boots and put on a tie, and he hoped this job at Farm Bureau would bring him that. So he said yes.

On the day we moved to Lumberton, I walked around the yard, sucking my thumb, saying, "I want to go home."

Momma said, "So do I, honey. So do I."

SCOTT

> *What I am interested in seeing you do is:*
> *sharing your food with the hungry,*
> *inviting the homeless poor into your homes,*
> *putting clothes on the shivering ill-clad,*
> *being available to your own families.*
> —Isaiah 58:6

I'M GUESSING THAT'S WHAT SCOTT'S MOTHER, MARY, said to him when they found the eviction notice on the front door of their apartment one August afternoon, when Scott was three years old: "I want to go home." Instead, they moved in with Mary's father. The father who had molested Mary since she was a small child. The father who continued to trade sex for rent.

I imagined Scott lying in his crib, listening to his mother's muffled cries; every neuron, every muscle, vibrating with the violation of his mother's body. Soon, they moved into a shelter. But to stay there, his mom had to apply for jobs and remain drug-free. She didn't like leaving Scott with strangers, knowing so well about abuse. She wanted something different for him, but couldn't remain drug-free, and when her drug screen came back positive, she was asked to leave.

A man came into her life, one who promised to take care of both her and her child. She quickly packed their few belongings into a suitcase and moved out of the shelter and into his home. The man failed to keep his promises, and it didn't take long before her drug use led to prostitution. Mary was threatened and beaten when she didn't turn enough tricks. Scott was left with whomever was around, while Mary worked and took drugs.

It's easy to say I would never do crack, or prostitute myself, or leave my baby with a pimp. That's simple to say if you have never lived a life of desperation and abuse, a life full of deprivation.

By the time Scott was five, he was so aggressive that the school mandated a psychiatric evaluation. That was when we met. And now, Scott had two brothers and a sister. Each time Mary got pregnant, her narcissism led her to fantasize that this baby would save her from another abusive relationship or the next eviction notice. But that never happened. Instead, the chaos grew. Their last eviction created homelessness for five.

The county offered temporary foster care placement for the children, but this terrified Mary. As incapable as she was at providing for her family, she was more afraid of strangers caring for her children. To prevent what she saw as the worst from happening, Mary set the apartment on fire. The flames screamed her anger and powerlessness. If her children couldn't live with her, they were better off dead. Their blackened belongings smoldered as the children were taken to the hospital to be treated for smoke inhalation. Now, foster care was mandatory.

> *Scott and his siblings purchased not love,*
> *especially not motherly love.*
> *God knows that nearly killed them all.*
>
> *But recovering from the fire*
> *that set the house to burn,*
> *match lit to turn to ashes,*
> *dreams of a room with a bed*
> *and a fuck from a friend.*
>
> *Burns now scarred permanently.*
> *Scott needed a place to live,*
> *so the search began for a foster home.*

*He was not suitable for younger siblings
since he knew only sexual connections;
touching and sucking were as natural
as hopscotch and jacks.*

*Social Services searched for a room
and a mom who didn't burn houses down
around her children while they slept.*

*Scott needed fostering care,
shelter and freedom from nightmares
of being on fire again.*

LUMBERTON, NORTH CAROLINA

Forgiveness is vital to our emotional health and spiritual survival. Without forgiveness, the family becomes a theater of conflict and a bastion of grievances. Without forgiveness, the family becomes sick.

—Pope Francis

AFTER DROPPING ME OFF AT TINY TOTS EACH MORNING before crossing the street to work, Momma managed the insurance office, an accountant by trade. She ran the business and our family with firmness. Customers appreciated Miss Dot and came to pay their bills in person instead of mailing checks so they could visit.

The first insurance agency was a one-room, wood-frame house in the parking lot of the Piggly Wiggly. When I was sick, I sat in the office on a folding chair, or lay on a cot, eavesdropping. Somebody's son died from swerving off the road to avoid hitting a pig. A preacher invited us to a church homecoming. Another customer asked for extra time on their bill.

Momma and Daddy extended credit to their customers, even when they were having problems paying their own bills. And Momma vowed, "Never will I complain about paying taxes if we ever make enough money to do so." I don't remember being poor, because I was young and there was always so much love and food: chicken salad, green beans, fried chicken, country-style steak, ham, butterbeans, black-eyed peas, candied sweet potatoes, corn and biscuits with sweet tea—gallons and gallons of sugar water soaked in Lipton tea bags, thick like syrup.

My parents gave the best customer service in town, and the business grew. After riding with Daddy to farms in the country to assess hailstorm damage, we consoled broken men who stood quietly beside ruined fields. They were thinking only two things: how to pay the bills that winter, and what crops would yield next year. Daddy was a comfort to them with his knowledge of farming. Because of his generosity, they never had to worry about their insurance lapsing. Momma and Daddy stood in agreement on that.

Folks socialized at the beauty parlor on Friday mornings at 9:30 a.m., with Momma. They knew when she got her hair washed and curled, and also knew it was the one time they could catch her sitting down—a good time to conduct business for the church, for the Daughters of the American Revolution, for her book or garden clubs. After I grew up and moved away, I went with Momma to get her hair done when I visited, relishing the goings-on in her beauty parlor.

Wanting to give us things they had to grow up without, Momma and Daddy made many sacrifices to make that happen. Although we never lacked necessities, toys, and especially life-size dolls, were scarce, until one day Daddy opened the trunk of his sky-blue Ford sedan and pulled a huge doll out of the trunk. My breath left when he took her gently out of the box and showed me how to hold her hand, pressing down hard on her arm so she could walk beside me. I loved Daddy and that doll. I named her Kathy, and we were inseparable. I treasured Kathy and protected her fiercely.

There was a rhythm to our lives that was reassuring, and although my parents worked six days a week, we ate supper together every day at 5:00 p.m. You could set your watch by the regularity with which we sat down to eat.

JANET

As long as you keep secrets and suppress information, you are fundamentally at war with yourself....The critical issue is allowing yourself to know what you know. That takes an enormous amount of courage.

—Bessel A. van der Kolk,
The Body Keeps the Score

JANET GREW UP WITHOUT MANY TOYS, TOO. But unlike me, she also grew up without affection. I remember the day she came to my office: the branches outside my window sent leaves cascading in an orange-gold dance. The beauty of fall's transformation caught in my throat, and it was in this blaze that Janet came asking for help, shortly after her forty-seventh birthday. Her story proved as memorable as the day.

Panic attacks were so frequent and debilitating that she rarely left the house. Suffering from anxiety since elementary school, now she could not function.

"Dr. Burns, I got your name from my nurse practitioner. She thinks you can help me."

Typically, I ask patients if it's an emergency or if can they wait a few weeks for an appointment. Janet, not wanting to seem needy, assured me she could wait. Her psychiatric evaluation revealed otherwise: generalized fear had increased into extreme anxiety. She distanced herself from her husband and children by reading science fiction novels and being ill. Migraines and mood swings created irritability and unpredictable angry outbursts. Initial and middle insomnia caused her to awaken in a panic, unable to breathe. Driving was particularly dangerous; panic attacks caused her to turn off the road. She felt as if she was going to die, and much of the time, she wished for death. The last attacks ended with her fingers curling and stiffening, a neurological event that occurs when breathing stops and toxins accumulate. By the time she came in, she was desperate. Her husband worked full-time and needed help with the household chores.

"Dr. Burns, if I even think about running errands, especially shopping, I am overcome with dread and paralysis."

Janet came from a broken family. Her mother, Rose, remarried when Janet was five years old, and shortly afterward, her stepfather began abusing Janet. Initially, Rose ignored the abuse, but eventually he enticed her to participate. One year later, Janet had a new brother, Bill. Janet's sexual abuse was frequent and painful. There was little love between family members, and lots of coercion. Choking and squirming against the pressure of abuse, she fought back at first, but soon resigned herself. In an effort to comfort each other, she and her brother began to be physical together, too.

The pressure to perform was relentless. They made good grades in school and were threatened continually not to tell about family relations. Bill ran away, sometimes making it to the train yard, where he would jump the train. Inevitably, his stepfather would catch him or he was returned by the police. He was beaten and threatened with worse violence if he disobeyed again. Bill continued to run away. Both children felt worthless and hopeless. They felt everything was their fault. When the parents' business declined, they lost their house and had to move in with the stepfather's brother. The physical and emotional torment worsened as the family's economic situation deteriorated.

Janet had group sexual encounters which her stepfather and step-uncle watched, participated in, or videotaped. Janet and Bill were often drugged during the filming sessions so they would be compliant. The family paid their bills and made extra money by selling child pornography. After many sessions with me, Janet grasped that she had been groomed for sex from an early age. She had no way of knowing it was wrong or that other children had different lives. Instead of doing math homework after supper, Janet and her brother taped a video. When sexual abuse was reviewed in health class, she did not connect the classroom version of abuse with what was happening to her. And even if she had recognized her abuse, she was easily constrained. Her parents, having been abused themselves, were well-versed in the art of manipulation. Janet's mother's role vacillated between that of silent observer and perpetrator. Janet remembers her mother mocking her when she complained. This contempt and disbelief caused much harm.

The sexualized relationships Janet had within her family violated normal boundaries and created fear and confusion. Denigrated, devalued, and violated, Janet had little chance of exposing the perpetrators. She had no authority to speak the truth, no one in her life who believed or loved her. Even so, she mourned the role she played in the abuse and felt deep shame about her behavior.

"It must have been my fault. I never said no, and sometimes if the touch was gentle, I enjoyed it. It was the only attention I got."

Trauma flourishes in environments where inappropriate and unsafe sexual boundary violations are repeatedly condoned or ignored. When authority and power are not equal in a relationship, there is no consent. The avalanche of resignations in Hollywood, television, the business and political world is representative of a paradigm shift regarding consensual sexual contact. This shift is necessary, and this revolution can only occur in an atmosphere of openness and compassion.

Janet often wondered why the school did not investigate

her frequent absences, her cuts and bruises. Why they ignored her vaginal bleeding, telling her mother that she "must have slipped on the swing," thus colluding with her mother. She wondered why the police never asked her brother why he kept running away before they returned him home for his beatings. At the time, societal norms protected perpetrators and isolated and shunned victims. Incest was unthinkable. Repulsed by the idea of a father who molested instead of nurtured, the truth was dismissed. The archetype of the nurturing father is programed into our DNA; our survival depended on it. But when abuse did happen, denial was injurious.

> *God made us lord over beasts,*
> *but a little lower than the angels.*
>
> *I pondered the truth of the message.*
>
> *Lord over beasts?*
>
> *Do they fornicate with their young?*
>
> *Do they beat, burn, starve, mutilate,*
> *and suffocate their loved ones?*
>
> *Lord, recreate us anew, like the animals*
> *we strive to be different from.*

It wasn't until Janet came to my office seeking treatment that she understood the impact of her traumatic childhood. Slowly unpacking her memories, she comprehended why the aroma of chocolate chip cookies caused a flashback and filled her with panic. Her keen sense of smell led her to remember her mother both as betrayer and baker, as cookies were used as a reward.

After months of therapy, she gained insight into the strange disembodiment and fear she felt while bathing and hugging her children, and gradually, as she remembered her abuse, she began to reengage with her family. Our work emphasized recovering memories and naming triggers that increased her anxiety, causing her to dissociate or "become fuzzy" in her thinking, fragmenting her behavior. Grounding techniques including breath work, yoga, and brain exercises allowed her to move from a reactive state to a calm nervous system. Together, we drew her nervous system, enhancing her understanding of her transition from safe calmness to fight-or-flight or frozen.

For many patients, the therapeutic relationship they forge with me is the first non-abusive relationship they have ever had. Fortunately for Janet, her husband was patient, understanding, and worked hard at breaking down destructive barriers in their communication. He attended several sessions, learning about PTSD, and began implementing verbal strategies at home which deescalated conflict and anxiety.

With encouragement, Janet's brother corroborated her memories, and gradually they pieced together the story of their childhoods. Before her stepfather died, she spoke with him and they remembered the life they had lived as perpetrator and victim. Her stepfather and mother took some responsibility for their actions, although they continued to minimize the abuse. Will the circle be broken by Janet and Bill's children? Not without therapy and safeguards, but I pray each day for transformation.

After months of treatment, Janet started driving again. Being able to shop without leaving her full cart abandoned in the aisles brought confidence, and slowly she began participating in her family's lives, going to sporting events and band concerts. Janet found a church family and started worshipping, accompanied by her husband and children. They found prayer and meditation to be a new modality for healing, one that did not require words. She now sells clothes in a boutique, enjoys the extra income, and is beginning to forge friendships.

The painting she created of a torn mattress lying on a basement floor, with a plate of cookies lying beside it, became a symbol of victory. As she reclaimed her breath and belief in herself by naming, mourning, and ultimately forgiving the violence that defined her childhood, it slowly lost power over her.

THANK THE LORD FOR THE NIGHTTIME

Praise with a blast from the trumpet,
praise by strumming soft strings;
Praise him with castanets and dance,
praise him with banjo and flute;
Praise him with cymbals and big bass drum,
praise him with fiddles and mandolin.

—Psalm 150

OUR GREEN ASBESTOS RANCH HAD TWO BEDROOMS with a den situated between. The house sat on a dead-end street, perfect for outdoor games—kickball and hide and seek. We had the best yard because of that dead end: no cars to watch for when we ran in the street. After scrambling to finish homework and change into play clothes, we gathered on foot, bike, or scooter at the corner of 26th Street and Barker. Red birds sang at that end of our street, right above the purple irises Momma planted and are blooming there still. Many times I've painted that red bird singing on the dead end sign, and I've never forgotten those trill notes or the cardinal's early teaching that the red bird sings loud and often when things seem the most bleak—either at a physical death, or the dead end I reached as Medical Director.

Since Momma worked outside the home, we had freedom from rules and prying eyes and all the sweets the kitchen had to offer.

> *I remember myself as a little light, white girl*
> *sitting on a tractor tire with my sister Penny,*
> *dredging troughs of water in the sand,*
> *while Momma shelled butterbeans.*
> *Southern yards sigh long into August, burning*
> *in the late cramping heat of summer's fever.*
> *Our red clay birthed bushels of beans, and*
> *Momma's shelling, peeling back taut green hulls,*
> *and popping pale, creamy beans*
> *into her white enamel basin*
> *forming the sounds of summer.*
> *See the sand shifting and slipping*
> *between our brown legs?*
> *Brown as Indians is what they called us,*
> *way before anyone thought of sunscreen,*
> *way before we worried about offending*
> *the Lumbee Indians*
> *by talking that way about dark skin.*
> *Dig, pat, pour, we were taking turns as we scooted*
> *to the faucet hiding under the nandina bushes,*
> *the ones Miss Connie called ugly.*
> *Daddy covered their roots,*
> *fighting winter's freeze and summer's drought.*
> *Skipping, jumping, slipping, as a green hose*
> *spurted rain toward our castles,*
> *and we flooded the swimming pool*
> *by the Mountain Dew man's house.*
> *"Let's make these waters whole," we sang.*
> *I can still hear two sisters giggling*
> *through the evening's bath,*
> *rubbing our hands over Ivory soap,*

pressing them in a prayer.
Opening our fingers just a crack and blowing,
wishing for a bigger bubble next time.
Later, lying together in a pink flowered room,
ironed sheets stuck to our skin
as salty sweat trickled down.

Sheer curtains bobbed
against a pine-framed window,
and we lay in bed, gazing at the backyard,
where the afternoon's shelling
and shifting had just dwelt.

When the black tires of our blue Ford crooned on the way to the tobacco fields where our parents grew up, Daddy's voice filled the car with songs. My favorite was "Chattanooga Shoe-Shine Boy." As Daddy belted it out, we bounced in the back, then leaned over the leather seat to peck him on the cheek with a kiss and begged him to sing it again. Sometimes he would sing another song or two, but it was never enough to satisfy his girls. Riding in our car, laughing for hours, no interruption existed except when we stopped to buy Nabs and a drink.

Daddy had a hard time picking out presents for Momma. Either he forgot a special occasion, or he got the wrong size and color. But one anniversary, we all hit the jackpot. Momma's present was a large stereo high-fidelity record cabinet. I can still see the delivery men trying to squeeze past the storm door to place it in the living room near the piano. Momma wasn't sure whether to be happy or mad. But Penny and I knew. We spent hours playing records on that hi-fi, our ears cocked to the music coming out of the speakers, discerning words to our favorite songs, writing them down so we could play them on the guitar and sing later.

"What did he say? *Thank the Lord for the nighttime?* Play it again, Penny." And she would, while Sue and Vivian, our best friends, scribbled furiously as I sang softly in the background, trying to catch the rhythm, the soul of the song. I knew the Lord had made the nighttime, and I knew I was grateful for it. But I wasn't sure exactly why Neil Diamond was, and I wanted to find out.

At the time, music was the extent of my sex education.

HARRY

> *If we look at this man's behaviors*
> *without knowing anything about his past,*
> *we might think he was mad.*
> *However, with a little history, we can see*
> *that his actions were a brilliant attempt*
> *to resolve a deep emotional scar.*
>
> —Peter Levine,
> *Healing Trauma*

SAFETY WAS FOUND IN THE TINY BEDROOM my sister and I shared, sleeping in a double bed, head-to-foot and foot to head. Sometimes our nighttime conversations got exuberant, and my father's footsteps stomped down the hall.

He opened the door and boomed, "If I have to come back here one more time, you're going to regret it."

We knew we would, and immediately lowered our voices to whispers. That kind of regret was something my sister and I avoided.

Another level of terror could transform a small child into a vicious, wild creature, almost unrecognizable as human. But I didn't know this until October 1997, when I interviewed Harry. The halls of the residential treatment facility at White Pines vibrated with tension that day because we were interviewing this aggressive juvenile delinquent. Harry had been kicked out of several psychiatric facilities and refused treatment in a half-dozen others. At age thirteen, living in a maximum security center in Montana, Harry was imprisoned. He repeatedly bit, kicked, or spit his way into isolation. Finding a therapeutic foster home had proved impossible. The state was spending hundreds of thousands of dollars keeping him in an out-of-state treatment center and wanted our help.

As the newest residential treatment facility in the state of New Hampshire, we were asked to take custody of Harry. Madeline, the clinical director, and I did not know much about him, and the details of his physical attacks on staff were unclear. We were interviewing Harry because the Office of Mental Health prioritized returning wards of the state closer to home, and therefore asked us to assess him. We agreed.

No patient had ever hurt me, and that was a source of pride. I knew that aggression proceeded fear, and this meant that I never threatened a patient, never approached patients in a domineering manner. Believing that my calm and mild demeanor created a safe environment for patients and myself, I was determined to keep it that way.

Just a few days ago, another patient, Helen, became so impatient with the treatment team's decision about her behavioral level that she kicked a hole in my door, her foot just a few inches from my head. Laughing loudly, she turned and ran down the hall, bragging to her peers that she had tried to kick Dr. Burns.

"I got her door, that bitch," she yelled, bragging about the hole she had left below my name plate.

While pondering this narrow escape, I heard the doors to the residential treatment facility (RTF) open and a security guard check in with Nicole, our receptionist.

"Dr. Burns, he's big. You better have someone in there with you." She rang my office to let me know Harry had arrived.

After walking down the hall, into the lobby to introduce myself, I looked and spoke only to Harry. He lifted his head and menacingly glanced my way, struggling to stand because he was shackled at the wrists, ankles, and waist. The security officers escorted him into my office.

"Please unlock the handcuffs and ankle chains," I said to the guards.

Reluctantly, they did, shaking their heads. And for the first and only time during my tenure as a child psychiatrist, security officers were placed at both doors of my office. The entire staff was on alert. Harry was well-aware that they were positioned outside the doors, but was more than confident that he could run or fight and there would be little anyone could do to stop him.

After swaggering into the office, he asked for something to drink.

"Would you rather have water or soda?" I asked.

"Soda." he answered, and drank thirstily when Cynthia, the charge nurse, brought it.

"I'll be listening, Dr. Burns," she said. "Just shout if you need anything."

Harry sought to intimidate with every movement. Eventually, when he saw that I was not going to react, he lay on the sofa. Looking up, he kicked off his shoes and threw them, purposefully missing my head.

That's twice this week that I've dodged a shoe. I silently gave thanks for my safety, and lowered myself to the floor.

Looking up at him, I decided not to ask questions, despite my curiosity. From his records, I knew Harry was an only child and his parents had divorced when he was two years old. Both parents neglected and abused him. Social Services had investigated the family more than forty times. As young as three, he was outside wandering and was found dirty and begging for food. He rarely came to school. When he did attend school, he had welts on his body.

Once, he presented with hundreds of cigarette burns. He told his case worker that a friend of his Mom's had tied him to his bed with duct tape, and raped him. Physical exams documented rectal bleeding and anal tears. Typically, exams of sexually abused children are within normal limits, making it difficult for pediatricians to substantiate abuse allegations. In Harry's case, the abuse was so aggressive, physical findings consistent with trauma were documented. In addition to severe aggression, his mental status exam showed that he feared adults, had chronic nightmares and anxiety. Other signs consistent with trauma included hyperarousal, flashbacks, dissociation, and emotional numbing.

Too few had studied his medical record, or they would never have threatened him or intimidated him into obedience. I decided to stay on the floor, about five feet from the sofa, and pray. *What can I possibly say to make him feel safe? How can I persuade him that our facility is different, that he can go to school, play soccer, or watch movies? That with us, he will not be raped?*

We rested there over an hour. He was exhausted from his trip, flying across the country in wrist and ankle chains, having to ask permission to speak, go to the bathroom, or eat. Eventually, he fell asleep, but I stayed awake, watching him, making sure that my head and body were low and nonthreatening. Each time he shuddered awake and startled because he did not remember where he was, I was there, quietly watching and waiting.

"You are here, Harry." I murmured while he slept. "Here with us. I'm your new doctor, and we are going to start over. You are the chairperson of your treatment plan. If you can stay safe, you will never go in the time-out room again. I pray that you find some peace here."

Although few words were spoken, Harry understood that he had entered into a different place, a place of respect and tolerance. We signed off on his admission papers so he did not have to be transported back to Montana. He was given a tour of his bedroom, the dining room, and the recreation room. His smile grew when he saw the Nintendo and learned that he was allowed to play video games before supper. The security guards left and took their chains with them.

The standard for our treatment facility was for all staff to approach patients in a quiet, neutral manner, and everyone knew the price to be paid if we lost a challenge. We quickly deduced that Harry's oppositional behavior was fueled by authoritative commands—answering confrontation with aggression. The staff understood that his rage was a cover for the fears created from years of neglect and abuse that he did not remember consciously, but his body had stored neurologically. That is why we never provoked patients or attempted to restrain them unless they were hurting themselves or someone else. Gradually, Harry responded to our therapeutic approach, and although there continued to be episodes that led to the time-out room, they lessened in frequency and intensity.

We listened. We helped him stay safe, and created an environment different from his home in as many ways as we could. Slowly, Harry began playing soccer more as his trips to the time-out room decreased. This is how we sang our success:

> *The boy was too difficult*
> *to be alone for the interview,*
> *so guards monitored the exam.*
>
> *Did he hear voices, or was he just a bad,*
> *mean, angry, devil boy?*
>
> *Pushing his way into our padded cell,*
> *banging his head on the vinyl,*
> *he ripped the fabric, splitting it and*
> *spitting on us, our facility,*
> *and his treatment plan.*
>
> *Anger poured from his memories,*
> *his butchered body and slaughtered soul.*
>
> *Not knowing how to live without the beatings,*
> *he brings his own pain*
> *now that he no longer lives with his mom.*
>
> *Surveillance was needed in the beginning.*
> *I was too late.*
>
> *The big burly monster that the father created*
> *when he raped the baby spit back at the world*

all the cum he had swallowed,
in his rage to forget the abuse.

He broke his head and our hearts
in the padded cell we created.

We built the facility to treat his disorder,
but he kicked us and dared us to care,
to cure him, so he could forget.

I remember ducking the spit
from the brave little boy.

He remembers the beatings and the rapes.

We should all remember this now,
for if he forgets,
who will remember?

LINDA

*On the night he shot his daughter, Linda,
I was walking with mine
on the pine-knolled shores of our beach.*

*The moon—shy, reserved at the outset—
shed her shadows, and reluctant no longer,
illumined a path lying easy on the ocean's surface,
lapping teasingly at our footprints,
rolling them away.*

*Two weeks before, a frightened mother had asked
a judge for temporary custody.*

*She asked because her husband threatened to
kidnap Linda.*

*He did this in front of the court house,
in broad daylight.*

He grabbed the mom, shaking and shaking her.

*Linda wept as an impartial judge said no,
granting the mother her restraining order,
but no protection for a little girl.*

And now she is dead. The life she had is gone.

*See us dancing on the dunes,
racing backwards in the sand,*

*while a bright planet emerges
and a red halo holds the moon.*

*Is that her night star shining fire on us
and on this mourning?*

*Red traces, light white spaces.
Can Linda see our black lab Pumpkin
chasing waves as my husband sits home reading,
worrying whether we were safe, wondering if we
will come home to him this night?*

*Far away, another mother sits alone,
not wondering when her daughter will return,
not worrying this night if she is safe.*

Still, that red halo wraps the moon.

If we all gaze upward, we can see this.

I READ THIS ACCOUNT OF LINDA in the local newspaper, verifying my dismay that no one wanted to see, hear, or touch abuse, and now another child had died. Who was gazing upwards, I sang?

PERFECTION

*There's not one totally good person on earth,
not one who is truly pure and sinless.*
—Ecclesiastes 7:20

PENNY AND I SLEPT TOGETHER in a double bed until I was ten years old. That intimacy forced us to lie with each other, confiding the day's adventures. No one had air conditioning back then, and our bedroom was just large enough to hold the bed, so we lay beside our pine-framed windows in the heat of summer, trying to catch a breath of cool night air.

She disliked sleeping with me; the lack of privacy drove her mad, and I wore leg braces. Those braces were a dangerous weapon when slung about in my sleep. Diagnosed as "pigeon-toed" by a pediatrician and an overzealous orthopedic surgeon, for years I was treated with braces, day and night, for *metatarsus varus*.

The daytime version of those braces consisted of straps that ran up my legs and hooked onto a belt around my waist, under my dress. Momma had to buckle me in while I stood still on the vanity stool. The nighttime version was the horror. A steel bar connected heavy brown shoes, so I had to lie on my back, toes pointing up and out in an attempt to correct in-toeing. I hated the confinement of that steel, but as with many childhood wounds, my memories vacillate between sharp and vague. I remember not liking it, but I don't remember my friends ever talking about it or teasing me. I could run fast, with or without braces, and was always picked for sports teams—maybe not first, but never last.

When I become a doctor, I realized how naive these treatments were. Understanding the anatomy of the leg reveals that the inversion would return as soon as the braces were taken off. Wrapping a six-year-old with elastic straps by day, and shackling her at night with a steel bar, was probably never therapeutic.

"You better not kick me with those things tonight, girl!" my sister said. "I'm warning you."

She wielded substantial power over me. Clinging tightly to my side of the bed, I stayed awake until I heard her breath even out and was sure it was safe to ease off, too. I never wanted to hurt anyone, especially her.

Penny and I had lessons in everything you can imagine. Sewing, ringing hand-bells, piano, choir, singing, etiquette, and dancing. Our parents wanted us to be perfect, and I still feel the mark of that. Even though Louise had just cleaned, vacuuming and dusting the den most Saturdays was required before we could go out to play. One "B" on our report cards was singled out, even among eight A's.

Betterment was Momma's desire, and I obeyed. My every thought was to make her happy. Penny rebelled, argued, and resisted. Her every thought was independence.

Each morning before school, she and I took turns practicing the piano for at least thirty minutes. One dressed while one played. Then we ate bacon, eggs, and grits swimming in grease and butter. After breakfast, we gathered our bookbags and walked the short block to school, petticoats rustling under our dresses, Mary Janes spit-polished, and white anklets with lace, folded neatly. No one else in my grade practiced piano before school, but Momma said it was "best to get it out of the way because you never know when something more fun is going to come along."

No, you don't, I thought, as I played my Mozart concerto one more time.

State auditions were next month.

On Saturdays, we played Snake in the Gutter with Momma after she had worked a half-day in the office, tallying up figures, paying bills, and listening to customers. She was always tired. When she wasn't working, she was volunteering—running for treasurer of the Garden Club or Daughters of the American Revolution, cooking or shopping for groceries, arranging the list at the church for office coverage, or talking on the telephone to a friend, helping them figure out some problem. Years later she was a founder of Meals on Wheels and a hospice volunteer.

She always made time for my favorite game, Snake in the Gutter, on Saturday, and it was a thrill to chase her down the cement walk that led to the front door. Standing in the middle while the other players ran across the sidewalk, the snake's job was to tag the runners.

"Got you, Momma. Now you're it!"

She was overweight, usually still in her work shoes, and easy to catch. Plus, I think she slowed down on purpose. I really loved her, so playing tag, cooking, or visiting folks after church was a tremendous joy. I did anything to get her attention, to stake a claim on her time.

Despite our parents' love for us, discipline in our home was harsh and frequent. We were spanked for disobeying—things like missing piano practice, not folding laundry, spilling our tea, and sometimes for laughing and whispering in church. These beatings were a constant threat, and they made us pull our pants down, a custom that intensified the shame and embarrassment. It also created a hierarchy of power and authority, which was not healthy, and which I deeply despised. And although our parents loved us, they enjoyed the intimidation they wielded. We were spanked with hands, belts, yardsticks, branches—any implement that could be turned into a weapon.

Most of my friends and cousins were spanked; we didn't share details, but I knew. It wasn't until later, after many years of psychiatric histories, that I realized how cruel our beatings were and how unnecessary. My momma said the dreaded, "This hurts me more than it hurts you," and, "Wait until your father gets home." The first I knew to be a malicious untruth, and it made me want to hurt them. You had to cry to make the beating stop, and that felt like a lie, too. Penny, stubborn as usual, would refuse, so that made it worse. The second, "Wait till your father gets home," was torture, as it gave you too much time to fear, because we knew what would happen as soon as we heard Daddy pull up.

My parents were locked in a fiery marriage. Imagine these beatings given in the context of their intense connection. Many mornings, sparks flew before I was up practicing the piano.

"Damn it, Dot. How many times do I have to tell you?"

And he had to tell her many times, because she was willful. Often correct, and always determined to get her way, Momma never backed down from a fight. Running the insurance business together was tough on their relationship. Momma was smart and capable. Her solutions to problems were often more practical than my father's, and he chafed against her opinions. They loved and depended on each other, but never settled into a calm marriage, and separated after almost forty years together.

Paddle round, river bend.

Flow that never ends,
continue into favored oceans.

Silt band rise from underneath and over, under
and over once more.

Winding knees of cropped cypress,
hanging moss, and copperheads.

Drift into and on my Lumber River.

Never ending gyration, cycle of paddles,
into twist and out, into twist and out.

Float downriver, dissolve into the black water
swamp that calls me home.
Into twist and out, into twist and out.
Reach inward flow, egress, become anew.
Washed river banks
searching for their way through the trees.

I didn't know then that I was the winding river bank, searching for my way. Telling about the beatings and the discord is not so you can judge my parents or pity me. I tell you because that punishment formed me. It made me afraid to be wrong. Striving for perfection and making sure I am good enough are engrained habits, even today, no matter how hard I've tried to purge them. Although not as violent as the abuse I treated in my patients, the quest for perfection was an unquiet and dangerous passage all its own, and left its mark.

Often, I say, "I was abused enough to be a good believer, but not so much that I can't do the work of listening and recording."

POST-TRAUMATIC STRESS DISORDER

*PTSD: the scientific initials applied
first to veterans who went to hell and back.*

*Bullets and bombs continue to shock
their neurological systems
in the grip of nightmares.*

*Helicopters drop shells every time a car backfires.
And we give the diagnosis initials,
proclaiming their disease an abnormal reaction
to the war they fought and everyone lost.*

*Armed for battle,
but not quite ready for the explosions
that would mark them forever as disordered,
now needing therapy and drugs
to exist in this world without tremors
and panic overtaking them.*

*Post-traumatic stress disorder,
a diagnosis for children?*

*Let's trace their reaction
when after a shower with Daddy,
they fight to the death not to ever use soap.*

*Ivory slipping and sliding over their genitals
before he did, making them dirty again.*

*They talk, they walk, they look just like children
who never knew war in their beds or bathtubs, yet
they battle each day for their lives.*

*And we give it initials, proclaiming a disease
that marks them as abnormal in the war
they are fighting and we are all losing.*

Post means after.

Traumatic means life-threatening wound.

*Stress means a physical force exerted
when one body part pushes on, pulls on, or
compresses and twists against another body part,
altering an existent equilibrium.*

THE SECRET

Nothing is covered up that will not be revealed, or hidden that will not be known.
—Luke 12:2 KJV

LIKE ALL FAMILIES, MINE HAD SECRETS. Daddy was too proud to admit any flaws, and hid both his blindness and his glass eye. We never talked about how he lost his vision until one day when I asked Momma and she told me this story: a chicken pecked Daddy near his eye, and then he got the measles. There was no saving his vision.

As little girls, we weren't allowed
in Daddy's bedroom or bathroom early,
before he placed his eye.
And even though we always traveled together—
four folks wedged in tight to a Ford,
two double beds at the Holiday Inn
—I never saw it out,
never saw the fleshy crater without its cover.
I don't remember exactly when
I was baptized with the knowledge,
entered the grownup world.
I do remember being ushered down the hall
by an older sister: carpeted roses

*led through an arch to the bathroom
and into the vanity, second drawer
from the left, the one in the middle,
to find a blue velvet box.*

*I don't remember what led to the discovery
of that glass marble eye,
rolling around on a red velvet cloth.*

*But I do remember staring, staring,
staring at the space in Daddy's head.*

*Wondering when the chicken that got him
was going to get me, too.*

*Wondering as I skipped down the street
to school, where that mad rooster had flown
after he pecked at Daddy's eye.*

*Wondering, wondering, wondering
what happens in the backyard when
you're little and a rooster eats your eye.*

*I remember wishing it hadn't happened
to Daddy—hoping my worry could
burn back the past, make it different,
ease that terror from our lives.*

*Figuring it must be my fault,
as I was the only one who shouldn't know about
the necromantic glass eye
hidden in the bathroom—
painted by an artist, vision of Daddy,
illustration of my childhood.*

Secrets work against children. They will assume that the reason they can't know is because somehow the problem is their fault.

I was no exception.

SALLY

There'll be no more stories of crime in your land,
no more robberies, no more vandalism.
You'll name your main street Salvation Way,
and install Praise Park at the center of town.
—Isaiah 60:18

CHILDREN PRACTICE BEING IN RELATIONSHIPS within their family, and they need innocent games in order to develop. Girls learn how to flirt by engaging their father's attention. Boys tease their siblings as they play, learning what is acceptable and what is bullying. This cannot occur if there are boundary violations within the family, especially sexual boundary violations. Without being able to trust the rhythms of family interactions—to play board games, kickball, to take turns setting the table so you can eat as a family—normal development is endangered. If your father never came home with a small gift that had no strings attached, then you do not know about consent.

When sexually abused children begin to date and explore intimate relationships, promiscuity and sexual connections are the norm. Peers' reactions to hyper-sexualized behavior range from shock and withdrawal to consent. But consent is not mutual if a child has been groomed for sex at a young age. Sexually abused teens quickly fall into the connections they know best, and their dating relationships advance physically before they can develop in other ways. This causes more trauma as interactions peak in intensity early, and then invariably fail.

Sally knew when she married her verbally abusive boyfriend at age twenty that she was making a mistake.

"Dr. Burns, I didn't love him. I was just so sick of my dad coming into my bedroom, so angry at my mother for turning away when he did, I accepted the first man who showed me attention. Boy, what a mistake that was."

After years of neglect and verbal abuse, Sally was able to free herself. She had three children and had been in the marriage for ten years, before seeking therapy. As she understood the role her father's molestation played, she was able to extract herself from her husband's abuse. Sally began to question her distorted view of herself, to understand that because she had lost her voice so young, saying no was difficult. However, she found her voice when the violence threatened her children.

"The last straw was when we were planting a garden and I said something casually, off-hand, that he didn't like. He reached out and broadsided me with the shovel. I thought, *If I don't get out of here, he's going to kill me or the children.* I left the next day."

DADA

*Bear with each other and forgive one another
if any of you has a grievance against someone.
Forgive as the Lord forgave you.*
       —Colossians 3:13 NIV

SATURDAY NIGHTS, WE WATCHED LAWRENCE WELK after eating steaks, baked potatoes, and salad with homemade dressing.

"Julia, you make the salad. Penny, you set the table and make the Thousand Island."

"Aw, I made the salad last week, Momma. It's Penny's turn," I said.

But once the chore had been handed down, it usually stuck.

Our love of food and music, mostly gospel and country, was intricately woven into our farming roots. The holiness of the earth rested in our blood, and Penny and I spent much time playing in the plowed fields of our grandparent's tobacco farms. Mud-soaked, hiding and seeking through mazes, we amused ourselves until supper. Never wanting to go inside, because that meant work—sweeping, dusting, setting the table. You better not say you were bored, because they'd give you something to do; keep you regretting those words forever.

I remember one day, riding out in the country, headed to Buckhorn. It could have stayed ordinary—the day, that is—because, like most days, it started out that way. Unexceptional in every manner: wake up, wash your face, brush your teeth so they shine. *Jesus wants me for a sunbeam to smile the whole day through.*

We rode in Daddy's car, winding through asphalt curves, swinging deeper and deeper into the country, where raindrops grow crops. Yields were going to be good this year. I heard the grownups talking late at night after I was supposed to be asleep. After sneaking out of bed and hiding in the kitchen, I peeped around the corner to eavesdrop. Good crops meant extra gifts at Christmas; maybe this year I could get a baton *and* a bike from Santa, instead of choosing between the two.

When we got to the house, our grandfather stepped out to greet us. My heart thrilled at the sight of this tall, lanky farmer who threw up his hand, waving as if we were best friends, forgotten to one another. Perhaps we were. It seemed that way to me as he beckoned us through the open front door, and we stepped into a living room bathed in streaks of white light, an oak brown rocker sitting in the middle. After climbing onto his lap, we ate M&Ms® without peanuts, and I marveled at the hollowed-out gaunt spaces his face held so deeply.

Knowing he was sick, I wondered if he could breathe his disease on me, if I could catch it and go with him to heaven. I didn't mind dying if it meant we could be together. At five years old, I was confident I could travel back and forth between worlds—eat M&Ms® after lunch with Dada and make it back in time to hold Michael, my best friend's hand in "A tisket a tasket, a green and yellow basket," for kindergarten recess. I didn't want to leave Michael, either.

After finishing my candy, I asked if I could go play. Nodding yes, Dada gently placed me on the floor beside his brass spittoon. A sprite, I bounced out the side door to find my cousins playing hopscotch, and after grabbing my pebble, I started hopping, too.

When I was a toddler, my grandfather and I played "Ride a horsey, ride a horsey down to town, take care of little Julia, don't let her fall down." While bouncing me on his knee, he'd open his legs wide so I'd fall through, and catch me just before I hit the floor. Then he grabbed me up, hugged me to his chest, and we'd laugh.

Today, that rocker sits in the corner of our den, waiting for grandchildren who are going to ride a horsey, too.

"Look at you, little Ju," he yelled, as he watched me hop.

Last week, my grandfather came in a dream to say that since time has more than one dimension, everything that ever happened was still present, both in the boards of his barns and in my paintings.

Fifty-two-by-forty-inch canvas recordings
of a little white girl's songs
so she can put them in a bucket,
take them to the beach,
and throw them in the ocean.

Let them float to the bottom
where the mermaids grow
—when they hear the stories they can tell, too.
It may not be much, but it is just enough.

The melodious chants of the auctioneer were a sad reminder of summer's end and the new school year's beginning. I held Daddy's hand as we listened to that humming, breathing in smells as the tobacco grader walked by, stroking golden leaves and signaling to the buyers.

I search the mirror for my father.
Shadows shade our living.

*Hidden memories are stirred
by a stray streak of farmland, red earth tilled
where straight furrows led to a barn.*

*Tobacco strung, leaves hung in threes on a stick,
weathered brown and aged.*

*Sticks lie drying in the heat,
hanging of summer's harvest and winter's goods.*

*Mules two-tied to a plow.
Daddy drove that furrow, topping green leaves,
wearing a Texas tie, boots, and glass eye.*

*Gazing at this memory, I wonder
what of me is his, and what is leftover
that I can claim as my own?*

*What remains after the suckering, the harvest,
after the long haul to market?*

*What price per pound does the auctioneer sing
today?*

SUNDAY SCHOOL

*When two of you get together
on anything at all on earth
and make a prayer of it,
my Father in heaven goes into action.
And when two or three of you
are together because of me,
you can be sure that I'll be there.*
—Matthew 18:18-20

MOMMA, PENNY, AND I DROVE A VAN around the county, picking up poor children, bringing them to Sunday School. After cookies and juice, we taught about Jesus, then they made art projects they could take home. I realize now those children came mostly for the snack and not for the lessons about God, but at the time, I had no concept of hunger. Feeling satisfied, walking the children to their front doors after Sunday School, one day I saw a tattered, dark living room filled with debris—uneaten food, dirty clothes, trash and torn furniture. Disbelief grabbed me. Anxiously running back to the van, I sat quietly in front with Momma. We headed home, where lunch was simmering—roast beef with carrots and onions.

    Like most safe and happy children, I believed that everyone's life was like mine and suffered when I learned that wasn't true. Praying that their dark and dirt would not attach itself to me, I never escorted another child to their front door, no matter how much Momma encouraged me. And I never told her why. I obsessed: why was my life blessed? Who gave the good life and who took it away? What kind of God delivered children so dirty and hungry to Sunday School that they couldn't go to church? Where were their parents when they walked out the door, and why didn't their mother spit on her finger and wipe off the smudges that blackened their cheeks?

While snacking on juice and cookies, those dirty-cheeked children learned they were precious in our eyes and God's. Praying daily for families to nurture children and protect them, for every person born to reach their full potential, these early experiences shaped a child-like faith that everyone is God's beloved, everyone deserves love. Many times, I have interceded for an aggressive or sexually provocative child in the school setting only to help the teacher gain new understanding. Parental neglect and aggression create disruptive, oppositional, and hyperactive children who become scapegoats, provoking further rejection and punishment. "Dr. Burns, I'll never forget what you've shown me about Susan's life. How her mistreatment and abuse caused her to be angry. How fearful she is that following my instructions will lead to more abuse. Thank you. I plan to change the way I interact with Susan."

Bessel Van Der Kolk, in his book *The Body Keeps the Score,* quotes Dr. Alan Sroufe, a researcher on maternal child attachment, as saying that resilience in adulthood can be predicted by one statistic: how mothers rated their kids at age two—loveable or unlovable. "By far the most important predictor of how well a child copes with life's inevitable disappointments is the level of security established with caregivers in the first two years of life." Mothers who rated their children as unlovable or demanding produced disruptive, aggressive children. If these same mothers are taught to soothe and love their children, the children become well-adjusted.[4,5,6]

CIRCLE OF LOVE

Her children respect and bless her;
her husband joins in with words of praise.
—Proverbs 31:28

QUESTIONS WITHOUT ANSWERS BECAME A SPECIALTY as my volunteering stretched beyond Sunday School: teaching adults to read, lifeguarding at a camp for mentally handicapped children, visiting the cancer institute to read the Bible or play the piano. Volunteer work allowed Momma, Penny, and me to be together. Our faith in God supported everything we did, inside church and out. Family was the other support, and six maternal aunts helped raise me. All worked outside the home as cooks, social workers, teachers, bank tellers, and textile supervisors, and each bestowed a different blessing. This circle of women, including Momma, my godmother, Agnes Julia, and Louise, our housekeeper and babysitter, created a tightly knit mantle of devotion. My Aunt Olive, was protector. When Momma and Daddy spanked me, I would call her and she would scold my parents, "Nobody better not spank my baby." It didn't matter that they didn't listen, but it did matter that she said it. On her next visit to Lumberton, she pretended to spank Momma for spanking me. I loved her for her gentle nature.

Our extended family's belief in each other and in God gave us a firm assurance that if we failed, something bigger backed us up. That *something* was larger, wiser, and kinder with mercy and grace flowing over. God never bickered with his sister or cheated by moving the timer down when he practiced piano. It was easy for me to be grateful, easy for me to feel God's closeness and his ability to protect. I was one of his chosen ones even if I couldn't figure out how you got chosen. "Jesus loves me, this I know," I sang happily, cutting construction paper and gluing bits to make a cross Momma could tape to the refrigerator.

After the closing prayer at church, we sang the Doxology as thoughts of fried chicken and caramel cake danced in my head. My aunts bustling in the kitchen as they cooked, I helped by setting the table or putting ice in the tea glasses. The food was delicious, and some days I miss that almost as much as I miss them.

Even now, there is a smell, say of hybrid tea roses,
that reaches me from the garden,
wafting through the house and lingering there
as I evolve into a little light white girl.

We are sitting in a parlor filled with roses,
eating tipsy cake on bone china.

These plates hold flowers
and this room holds all our wishes.

Momma dared her daughters to move through life
like the hybrid teas of the past,
with an old Southern style.

Sometimes I sit with my roses.

Sometimes I sit with my Momma
in a garden parlor, eating tipsy cake,
weaving a memory and sprouting wings
that rock me to and fro between these worlds
—the present and the long ago.

A NURTURING FAMILY

I think that was his tragedy—he didn't know what he was, and so he was nothing...that he didn't know what he was and there was no possible way in life for him to find out. Which to me is the worst possible condition a man could find himself in— not knowing what he is, and to know that he will never know.

—William Faulkner,
Light in August

WHEN OUR SON BENJAMIN WAS IN FOURTH GRADE, he was asked to write an essay describing the ideal nurturing family. A few years ago, I framed it and gave it to my husband for Father's Day. The necessary ingredients for families—respect, love, listening, discipline, faith, good deeds, chores, and fun, coupled with no bullying or hypocrisy—are outlined, succinctly with the occasional spelling woes of a third grader.

> *An ideal nurturing family is a family that respects one another and their opinions or thoughts. If they have a big change in the house, they will ask or vote before someone does it. They will not allow inappropriate movies. Each family should have a certain faith and go to church. They should spend*

time with their families. They could go on bike rides, fish, go out to eat, or play games (Monopoly), or you could play games outside (football). The kids should be in activities such as basketball, soccer, hockey, or skateboarding. Parents should have at least one kid. The parents should tell them to wear a helmet, don't say bad language, or make fun of people. Especially, parents should not be hypocrites by smoking or not wearing a helmet when biking; they must set a good example. They should be healthy and nice, but not if punishment is needed. Also, you should donate money, and the kids should help around the house. The end.

You can tell that the rules of a "good enough" family were engraved in his being. He did not create this essay out of his imagination, but out of his life, from the love and safety that surrounded him.

A beautiful eight-by-ten-inch photograph of Gray is in my bathroom: my baby girl when she was one month old, lying on a pink quilt made by her great-aunt Barbara, on top of that a gorgeous white knit blanket made by our namesake, Olive Gray. She is pulling on the bracelet I wore as a baby, and wearing a gold cross bought by her grandmother. All three of my children wore that christening dress and the beautiful crocheted bib with a blue ribbon. In this photo, you can tell she is loved. Already, she is gazing straight at the camera, her head thrown back, a big grin on her face, looking confident. Swaddled in clothing that a family member wore or made, she is almost suffocated in the traditions of two families.

I keep this photo on a shelf in our bathroom to remind me to lift her in prayer now that she is an adult:

Dear Lord, protect her, nourish her, embolden her to grow, renew her on her magnificent journey. Help me to be grateful for her independence as she grows away from us. Allow me to revel in her spirit of adventure while she studies abroad.

It is difficult for me to have these loving memories of my daughter without comparing them to a patient I saw recently. Alan was being seen for aggressive behavior in school and at home. He swore and threatened his mother, teachers, and peers. Truant so frequently, he was at risk of incarceration and had been referred by the courts in an effort to keep him at home.

"What's your proper last name, Alan?" I ask him, confused, seeing that the last name he used was not the last name on his chart.

Prescriptions have to be written in a precise format, and proper names are not optional.

"I go by both," he replies.

"Which name do you want on the prescription? Your legal name?"

"It doesn't matter."

Doesn't matter? How can it be that your name does not matter?

"It matters," I say. "It matters to me."

"Well, Dr. B., I just don't know. Folks call me both."

How can you put your life into context without belonging to a family and knowing your name? How do you establish what and who you are? Alan and Gray both demonstrate, in opposite ways, the necessity of good-enough parenting. Brought into the world to create a portrait of their walk on earth, one child is given all the brushes, paint, and canvas she needs to establish her own identity. The other is not given a name. And we wonder at their outcomes. One at risk for incarceration, with a rap sheet. The other on scholarship, studying to become a doctor.

Next time you look in the mirror, ask yourself if you know your name. If you do, be glad and generous. There are children out there who don't.

STEVE

As long as you keep secrets and suppress information, you are fundamentally at war with yourself...
—Bessel A. van der Kolk

SEXUAL ABUSE COMES IN A VARIETY OF FLAVORS, and sometimes does not involve physical contact. Such was the case with Steve, who came in on a court order. He had violated his child-custody agreement, and if he wanted to continue seeing his son, he had to have therapy. Rarely do I take court-ordered cases, because the motivation for change is low. Patients typically are compliant only to fulfill their mandate. But I had seen Steve several times before he confessed that his treatment was mandatory, and I was reluctant to dismiss him.

As far back as he could remember, Steve was exposed to pornography. His father was addicted and frequently left his magazines and pictures out so Steve could see. Initially, Steve found them when his father was absent. Gradually, it became an activity they did together. Steve had no idea this was wrong. He had no thoughts of stopping. He had a vague notion that his father would get aroused when they looked at the pictures. He was sure that his father never physically molested him or asked Steve to touch him, but their viewing sessions in the garage were frequent.

When Steve married, he chose a woman who had been sexually abused. Molested at age fourteen, Priscilla remembered making-out in the music minister's home while his wife rested upstairs. As a result, Priscilla chose a series of older men who physically resembled her perpetrator. She would bring them home, and they would "watch a movie" while her husband was working. Priscilla felt extremely guilty allowing Steve to use Priscilla's infidelity as an excuse to continue viewing pornography. Online hookup sites stimulated him, and evenings were dedicated to porn while he said he was in the home office "doing paperwork." Family time suffered.

One day, when Priscilla was cleaning the home office, she clicked on the computer and several pornographic sites popped up. Some contained photos, but others were dating sites. A Share Your Wife site popped up with her own naked photos. Priscilla confronted Steve, and he admitted to looking at pornography and posting her photos. He denied hooking up, but for Priscilla it was the end. She had to leave. They had been working on his pornography addiction in group and couples therapy for years, and she felt this betrayal deeply. She left that week and filed for divorce.

In the separation agreement, counseling was required so child visitation could be unsupervised. Unfortunately, Steve was not motivated. He did not fully disclose his online dating hookups or the amount of time he spent looking at pornography. A referral to a sex addiction group was made, and he went sporadically but was never invested. His son continued to visit on weekends. The child's safety was not certain.

Priscilla engaged in therapy and began to discover why she had married a man with a sex addiction. Why she engaged in heavy petting with other men. Her curiosity brought one revelation after another regarding her compulsions and coping mechanisms. The impact that abuse had on her life was gradually revealed as she stayed in therapy, determined for her son to have a life free of addictions. Steve was making that difficult because his obsession with pornography dictated his life, leaving little time to spend with his son, who was likely to absorb his lessons about pornography, even without shared viewing sessions.

CHESTNUT STREET METHODIST

> *Do you not know that your bodies*
> *are temples of the Holy Spirit, who is in you,*
> *whom you have received from God?*
> *You are not your own.*
> —1 Corinthians 6:19 NIV

IN LUMBERTON, THERE WAS SCHOOL and there was church, with little else in between. Our church, Chestnut Street United Methodist, was a constant in my life. Momma pinned curlers in our hair on Saturday nights so it would fall perfectly on Sunday morning. During worship, I looked pretty while memorizing the books of the Bible frontwards and backwards, shouting out answers in our Bible drills. My preferred place to be at 11:00 a.m. on Sunday was in our pew, resting my head on Momma's shoulder or sitting beside Daddy, sometimes pinching my sister for the best seat, and getting pinched back.

"*I got the joy, joy, joy, joy down in my heart,*" I hummed, as I buzzed around the house.

When other teens were listening to the Grateful Dead or Led Zeppelin, I was singing hymns in the youth choir and ringing hand bells.

Wednesday night services were a good time to go to the altar and claim Jesus—get saved. Sometimes you felt something stirring deep in your soul. Sometimes you went because your Momma nudged you, or you looked out of the corner of your eye as your best friend eased her way up. You didn't want to get left out; if she was going to heaven, you wanted to go, too.

Chestnut Street Church was where I wanted to be, because there was little else to do in this sleepy Southern town. Church was the main activity. We had a Methodist youth center with pool and ping pong. Whoever you were dating would join, so it was a good way to be with your boyfriend without it counting as a date. Sometimes girls sneaked out the back and left, but they usually got caught. Either their parents came to pick them up early and found them gone, or their hickeys gave them away.

One day after church, Daddy told Penny and me that he wanted to talk to us separately in the living room. The living room was saved for company and discipline, so neither of us was excited about the prospect of having an appointment there. Both he and Momma were sitting down. I sat also. Then Daddy asked me if I thought Ray, a junior in high school, and Suzy, our much older and married youth director, were involved.

"How?" I said. "What do you mean involved?"

"Are they boyfriend and girlfriend?" he asked.

We had just been on a youth retreat, camping by the lake, singing songs, making fires, and cooking campfire stew. It was a Holy-Spirit-filled week, and so, incredulous at the suggestion, I said, firmly and resolutely, "No."

"Are you sure?" he asked.

Daddy was president of the council and wanted to know how to lead the congregation through this. Either it was a scandal, or it was a scandalous lie.

"Absolutely, Daddy, I'm sure. I just spent the week with them. I think I'd know if something was going on."

The next week, Suzy left her husband, moved out of her apartment, and the affair I was sure couldn't be, was public. Later, she and Ray married, had children, and a good life together.

I didn't see it then as anything but love, an accident that

couldn't be prevented. Clearly, there were boundary violations, but since she was a woman, it was easier for most folks to look the other way, even though she was an authority figure and a church leader. Some people found it hard to understand and left Chestnut Street, questioning their faith in this incident where God was found wanting through a minister's behavior. Some moved to the Presbyterian Church. Some decided to become Baptists, and others simply stayed home on Sunday mornings. This early encounter with inappropriate sexual boundaries shocked me, but at the time, I didn't understand them fully.

It was years before I realized how frequently church leaders confuse the rapture they feel for the Lord as something to look for in another human—wandering into an out-of-bounds sexual relationship that fails to satisfy; yet another human relationship that disappoints.

Folks didn't discuss it much after they left. There was a certain rule of hypocrisy that reigned in churches and homes: if you don't talk about it, it didn't happen. Or at least, it's not a problem.

The security I found in my family and church community developed my compassion, while the inequities I witnessed at church, school, or in my volunteer work dispelled some naiveté. Mostly, God was good to me and I was good to him. Kneeling each night by my bed, I thanked God for my life and for the people in it who loved me.

"God bless Momma and Daddy, Penny and Aunt Olive…" And I implored him, "Help Suzy and Ray stay together in true love, because they have made so many people unhappy. Make Penny give me a ride to school without fussing, and if I should die before I wake, I pray the Lord my soul to take. And Martha B. can have Joseph. I don't care about him anymore, God, even if he is good about checking the weather every night. I can do that by myself. Amen."

I never thought I would die, though. That God would ever come after my soul and take it.

PETER

The ACE (Adverse Childhood Experiences) Study has shown that child abuse and neglect are the most preventable causes of drug and alcohol abuse, mental illness, unwanted pregnancy, divorce, domestic violence, incarceration, and they are a significant contributor to the leading causes of death, such as diabetes, heart disease, cancer, stroke, skeletal fractures, liver disease, and suicide.[7]
—Julia W. Burns, MD

OUR CARPENTER, PETER, WAS BUILDING a porch on our house when an emergency call came from the residential treatment facility. He was listening when I gave an order for stat medication to subdue a resident, Eddie, who was cowering in the time-out room and kicking anyone who came close. After recommending that they monitor his arousal and mood while supporting his post-traumatic stress disorder with relaxation techniques, I hung up.

The phone call jolted Peter, and several days later he said, "Remember when you were talking to the hospital and I was working on the porch? Well, it brought up some things I hadn't thought about in years. It happened to me, too. A man, Leon, tried to molest me when I was eleven. He was a friend of the family, and when my father died, he swooped in, preying on my brother and me. He knew what he was doing. He kept a lot of dirt bikes and four-wheelers, always inviting seven or eight boys over to his house. He enticed us, taking us fishing and camping. One night, I was over at his house and we were going camping, but no one else came. I asked him, 'Where are the other guys?' He told me they were going to meet us there. We got to the campsite, but as darkness came, none of the other boys joined us. There was no tent.

"Then he turned to me and said, 'We're going to sleep in the truck tonight.'

"As we settled into the cab of his truck, he began to grope me. He was feeling everywhere, and the blood rushed into my face. My heart was pounding, and my chest was so tight I could barely breathe. I was scared. I told him I had to pee and got out of the truck, thinking about how to get away. The main road was four to five miles off, down a gravel road, and then when you got to the main road it was a long, long way home. But I took off running until I heard his truck driving slowly down that gravel road after me. Every time he stopped, I stopped. He was listening for my footsteps, and I was breathing so loud I was sure he could hear me. When he started off, I ran like mad, so afraid he was going to catch me, and I didn't know what he would do. I just ran, doing all I could to get away.

"I was so ashamed. I felt filthy. I felt like it was my fault. I was afraid to tell my Mama—she would blame me. And if I couldn't tell Mama, who could I tell? Who would believe? I kept it inside. I stopped going to that man's house, but my brother kept going. I stayed away from my brother after that because I knew what was happening and I couldn't believe he would do that. I turned against him, and I think I regret that the most. He was about fourteen and I was eleven. I blamed him for not protecting me, for doing nasty things with Leon. I couldn't wait to grow up and get away from them all.

"As I grew, I became wild—drinking and using drugs. I was filled with hate. Staying up for days, I played cards and did drugs—methamphetamine, coke, any drug. I didn't care. Once I was strung out and I went fishing with two friends. When we got to the river, it was high, so we tied our gear around our necks and tried to cross. I got swept away by the water while swimming. My feet were dragging, pulling me under. I was struggling to breathe, and the water roared over my head as I lifted my arms in one last effort to pray. Knowing I was dying, I wanted to ask forgiveness. I didn't want to go to hell, and that's where I thought I was headed. If the afterlife does last for eternity, I wanted something better than darkness.

"After stretching my arms out one more time, I felt something grab me. It was a root, and I slipped my hands through it and hung on for twenty minutes, my mouth and nose barely out of the water. While catching my breath, I gradually gained the strength to drag myself up on the bank.

"The next Sunday, I went to church. I couldn't wait to go, and, as I lifted my hands to thank God, a white light filled me with peace, and that day my heart turned from hate. I started talking in tongues, although I didn't know what that was. I'll never forget the day I was filled with the Holy Spirit.

"For years, I wanted to hurt him like he hurt us. But after being saved, I ran into Leon and just walked by him. Trying to live my life for God, I felt love for Leon. If I had seen him before I got saved, I would have killed him or hurt him bad.

"We've talked about it since, my brother and me. My brother had a hard life, serving years in jail for drugs and other stuff. Anger and violence destroyed him, and I was afraid when he got out of prison. But one day, a Pentecostal woman witnessed to him, and he came home, reading the Bible to Mama and me, telling us what he had learned. Since then, he's been faithful, a good father to his three boys.

"What do you think should happen to men like Leon?" Peter said.

I explained that there aren't enough prison bunks for molesters, so many men and women are perpetrators. Since the abused all too often become abusers, and often perpetrators are victims who have not had any intervention, the problem compounds and will continue unless safeguards are put in place. The Catholic Church and the Boy Scouts demonstrate this pattern.

"Perpetrators seek connection by touching children inappropriately," I told Peter, "and unless community-wide treatment and prevention programs are available, there is little hope that children will be safe. Children need protection, yes. And molesters need trauma treatment. But we can't help either while we pretend it isn't happening."

This answer didn't satisfy him. "I can tell you that if someone tried to molest my ten-year-old son, I'd have to deal with them. There wouldn't be enough room on Earth for both of us."

I nodded in understanding and asked if we could pray. Anointing him with holy oil, I asked the Lord to bless him and keep him, to make his face shine upon him and be gracious unto him, for the Lord to lift up his countenance upon him and give him peace. And then I spoke praise for the brave little boy who hurried down a gravel road forty-one years ago. Running in the dark, escaping the groping hands of a thirty-year-old man who drove beside him, bright lights shining into the trees that were shielding the boy from that destruction. I saw Jesus running in front, holding branches out of the way so that young boy could speed forward. I asked for forgiveness and mercy for his mother, who didn't know and couldn't protect her children. And then I asked a special blessing on the older brother, who has his own story, his own suffering.

After Peter finished his story, my husband told him, "This man, Leon, was most likely molested as a child. You have to believe this. Julia has convinced me."

But Peter refused to listen. Praying for Peter as I lay down to sleep that night, asking God to bring back forgiveness, I felt the weight of Peter's angry life, the drug addiction and alcoholism, the fractured relationships, and the lack of self-worth.

And this is a story with a happy ending. This child got away, but not without years of hard work and difficulties.

CAROLINA

*"I'm a Tarheel born, I'm a Tarheel bred
and when I die, I'm a Tarheel dead."*
—University of North Carolina,
Chapel Hill fight song

MY SENIOR YEAR IN HIGH SCHOOL, the admission director of the state university came to our school and said, "Put your name on the application, and if you sign it, have decent grades and SAT scores, you're in."

Surely his message was more complex, but that's how I remember it, and that's what I did. Robeson County didn't send many students to the University of North Carolina.

Nonchalant about college, I didn't apply until after Christmas, and it was my grades not my standardized scores that resulted in my acceptance. An audition in the music department led to my assignment to Fritz Wang's studio, and I headed to Chapel Hill to study piano that fall.

My father graduated from the rival agricultural college down the road, and threatened to put me on the bus because there was "no way I'm taking a traitor to that school." Of course, when moving day came, he and Momma loaded a borrowed truck and proudly drove me to Hinton-James, a new dorm on south campus.

Male students were everywhere, standing in elevators with their boxes as we rode to the eleventh floor. The floors were separated by gender, but it was unsettling. I was making my bunk when my roommate, Sherry, an African-American, entered with her parents. My parents were surprised, but they quickly gathered themselves and asked her family to join our picnic. There was more than enough food. I remember the picnic Momma packed—pimento cheese sandwiches, chicken salad and pickles, pound cake and ice box cookies—my last for months.

That night, students of Hinton-James gathered with the resident advisors for orientation. They gave us lists of resources, restaurant recommendations, maps of the campus, and a lecture on birth control. I'll never forget the demonstration they gave about condoms and diaphragms. I thought, *Well, if I have to do that, I'm going back home.* Luckily, sex turned out to be an elective that year.

When classes started, I learned about philosophy and women's studies. Reading about how women participated in the Civil War and the Underground Railroad, even as they were denied the right to vote, inspired me. There were not enough hours to practice piano, study, and learn. I felt the need to rush, to try to catch up, to know as much as my classmates seemed to know. Even now, I'm not sure what I was trying to seize, but I was running after it as fast as I could.

The message of the Methodist Church served me well until I went to college. But now, I wanted to drink a beer on Saturday and go to church on Sunday without being told I was going to hell. So I became an Episcopalian. I was smart enough to know I wanted beer and heaven, too, even if I wasn't so sure about sex.

I excelled in all classes except for music. Advanced Music Theory met three days a week at 10:00 a.m., and our professor, Mr. Boco, a short, balding Italian man, loved to scream and tap his baton. One morning, he sat on the piano bench and played five measures of a Bach fugue, and asked us to write it on staff paper.

I laughed. thinking, *What a good joke.*

Looking around, I saw students working, and stopped laughing. Since many classmates had written the composition correctly on their staff paper, I immediately sought assistance in dropping music theory. But when exams came, I discovered I was still enrolled in Advanced Music Theory 203. A clerical error caused me to take that final. That "C" kept me out of Phi Beta Kappa—the only fraternity I've ever desired to join—but I was glad to get it.

By my sophomore year, I had changed majors.

ADVANCED ABNORMAL PSYCHOLOGY

*Love one another.
In the same way I loved you,
you love one another.
This is how everyone will recognize
that you are my disciples
—when they see the love you have for each other.*
—John 13:34-35

AFTER DROPPING MUSIC, I CHOSE PSYCHOLOGY as my major. Two semesters of abnormal psychology allowed me to sign up for Advanced Abnormal Psychology, where we studied things with Dr. Carly that you'd never learn at Lumberton High.

During a class trip to Charlotte, we visited a transgender bar. You could cast a vote in the Cher look-alike contest.

"Are these men dressed like women, or are they women?" I asked my professor, wondering where I was headed, where the voyage from music to psychology was taking me.

The women looked so beautiful, so feminine.

"Hey, Julia, want a screwdriver?" Tricia yelled, from across the crowd.

"No, thanks!" I screamed back, over the heads of hundreds of transvestites.

Or were they transgender? Differentiating would be easy now, but I couldn't then. I chose not to drink that night even though I wasn't driving. I wanted to stay fully sober, to remember whether the winner of the Cher contest was wearing the black fishnet stockings or the red hat.

After meeting in a room behind the bar, a discussion was led by a transgender person who was moving to Canada for gender reassignment surgery. While reviewing life, how she dressed, and who she loved, she educated us. Even in our ignorance, the room was filled with compassion and little judgment. It wasn't difficult for me to know that God made everyone and loved them the way they were. My education about sexual stereotypes, sexual identity, and gender identity began in that small, smoky bar and continues every week in my office.

That spring, our class took another trip with Dr. Carly. This time, we went to a coal mining village in West Virginia, where we camped in a state park on Easter weekend so we could attend services at a small mountain church and witness snake handlers.

"They will pick up snakes with their hands; and when they drink deadly poison, it will not hurt them at all; they will place their hands on sick people, and they will get well" (Mark 16:18).

Having accepted an invitation to the preacher's house, we trod carefully over high grass in the backyard behind his brick rancher, where wooden boxes lay marked *Danger, Poisonous Snakes*.

"Be careful not to stick any fingers or toes too close to those wood boxes," our professor said. "There are rattlers, cottonmouths, and water moccasins in there."

There was no hospital nearby to wrap a tourniquet and inject anti-venom.

I carried rolls and rolls of black-and-white and color film, along with a new Pentax camera, and documented the miracles. Boldness led me to the altar, snakes writhing and wriggling so close I thought I could hear their tongues rolling out of their mouths. No background music played, because snake-handling, a hypnotic dance between man and reptile, required concentration. Women stood drinking strychnine out of mason jars.

    These people followed a literal translation of the Bible, and we witnessed this merging with the Holy Spirit in defiance of death. Survival was a language they spoke well, and we listened and believed, sitting in their pews.

    I still have those photos and pull them out once in a while, looking intently to see what was revealed the moment the shutter clicked, aperture wide open in the darkness of that country church. The men, shrunken and pummeled by coal mining, seemed larger than life and all-powerful as they stretched their hands into those crates; the women, supernatural as they tipped jars of poison to their mouths. I must have wanted to merge with the Holy Spirit, too, because I was close. You can tell from the angle of the camera that those snakes could have clamped a fang in my arm.

BIRTH OF A DOCTOR

No, we neither make nor save ourselves.
God does both the making and saving.
He creates each of us by Christ Jesus
to join him in the work he does,
the good work he has gotten ready for us to do,
work we had better be doing.
—Ephesians 2:10

THE DAY I DECIDED TO BECOME A DOCTOR, leaving piano and psychology behind, was during a psychiatric rotation at the state hospital: Advanced Abnormal Psychology, senior year. Every week, our class visited the acute ward, where new patients were admitted in the midst of a psychotic or manic episode. When we got to the unit, we had to ring a bell so nurses could come and unlock a thick wooden door, before we stepped in. If that sounds easy, it wasn't. Because often, acute psychosis patients were aggressive, heard voices, agitated, and often suicidal.

The hollow clang of the door locking behind us was a sound to which I never got accustomed. Hyper-religiosity, a common sign of mania, led me to meet many patients who thought they were Jesus. We read to patients, helped them write letters, organized belongings, or just sat with them.

Toward the end of the semester, we began assessment and diagnosis—interviewing a patient in front of our peers and professor. This process was nerve-wracking, and we spent long hours practicing interviews with each other. It was late winter when I conducted an interview with Sam, a patient in the ward. He and I walked into the exam room together. There I was, eager to learn, and he was old and twitchy, leaning hard right to hear voices inside his head that only he could hear.

As we sat in the metal chairs, he asked, "Do you want a candy bar?"

I said yes because I loved candy. I also wanted to break the ice, win him over.

He replied, "With or without nuts?" and began to belly laugh.

Joining in, our laughter merged into joy. Gratitude for my first patient continues—for the teaching and intimate sharing, for the good grade, but mostly for the laughter—and I've been living in laughter and tears with patients ever since.

After escorting patients back to the ward and returning to class, we discussed the diagnosis and treatment plan. As we were discussing each case—schizophrenia, bipolar disorder, and depression—I realized that most patients were taking two to three medications. Neither I nor my peers knew how medications affected the brain. How does serotonin and norepinephrine-receptor growth change with anti-depressants? Which anti-psychotics block dopamine without tardive dyskinesia, a movement disorder?

In that moment, I decided to apply to medical school, with only one lab science, zoology, on my transcript. I had taken this course on a dare from Penny, who thought I couldn't pass a science class. But it didn't matter. After checking in with Momma and God—probably in that order—I settled on my decision.

Since I had not taken pre-med classes, that fall I proceeded as planned with psychology graduate school at York University in Canada. As my master's thesis, I proposed the study of gender differences in language.

Research in clinical psychology was tedious and repetitive, so it wasn't long before I started applying to medical schools. I set my cap on McMaster, a Canadian school that accepted liberal arts majors, and offered a year-round program that could be completed within thirty-six months. Saving time by skipping the requisite pre-med courses appealed to me, so I applied and was granted an interview.

The day proved intriguing as a nun, a physicist, and a traditional pre-med student joined me for a two-hour ethics discussion observed from behind a one-way mirror. McMaster Medical School was committed to diversity and wanted only self-motivated students.

Captivated with the idea of studying medicine in this atmosphere, I spent the year dreaming of acceptance.

JEANNETTE

Everything was created through him;
nothing—not one thing!
—came into being without him.
What came into existence was Life,
and the Life was Light to live by.
The Life-Light blazed out of the darkness;
the darkness couldn't put it out.

—John 1:3-5

IT WAS A DIFFICULT SESSION, so after my patient Jeanette left, I went outside to clear my head. The New Hope Creek flowed by my office in Chapel Hill, and hovering over the water and rock beds, I consciously released any remnants of our interview.

"Cleanse me, Lord. If I have picked up any negativity, let me release it. Fill me with joy and love. Let me imagine this woman healed of her sexual molestation—the assault from her soccer coach that settled into her body, creating a dissociative and fragmented person. Give me strength to help her redeem this story, this rape that occurred for years as her coach drove her home after practice—her parents too busy to notice the failing grades and her hiding. Compassion, Lord. Love, Lord. Renewal and protection as she begins this process of remembering, and I this process of listening."

As a result of her sexual molestation, Jeanette became a silent observer as her son, Sam, sexually abused three of his siblings. Now the children were adults and were all suffering from chronic illnesses: autoimmune dysfunction, depression, and anxiety. Gender identity diffusion was present in several. Wounds were bleeding all around, and no one had named it or helped stop the hemorrhage.

Jeanette's children depended on her for housing and financial support. Finally, she decided that her paralyzing panic attacks and numbness were more than she could bear. On the first visit, I knew individual therapy would be minimally effective, so I referred her to family systems work and dialectical behavioral therapy. But she was afraid. Afraid to stay still, and afraid to move forward. Afraid to know, but paralyzed with the not knowing.

Jeanette deeply regretted the actions she and her husband had taken when their daughters revealed the abuse. Although they sought treatment for the girls individually, they never worked in therapy as a family, and they had not asked Sam to move out. Years later, anger and resentment threatened to tear the family apart. The brother, Sam, who had started molesting his sisters when he was thirteen and they were younger, had an apartment and a job, but now he was not allowed in the home. I felt certain that Sam had been abused prior to becoming a perpetrator.

"You don't start having sex with your sisters at age thirteen unless you have been exposed to sex, pornography, or have been abused," I repeated frequently.

Jeanette recounted a fundamentalist church that she and her young children had attended regularly. She told of how the Sunday School teacher had been accused of sexually molesting several children. There was no criminal investigation, and the church leaders refused to believe the accusations. The teacher was allowed to remain in his role, and the families making the allegations were shunned. Jeanette states that, at the time, she thought the church was correct, and continued to let the children go to Sunday School. Now she wondered if this was a possible source for Sam's abuse.

By the time she came to see me, Jeanette was prepared to do whatever it took to heal. She worked hard in therapy and committed to family therapy, which she made mandatory for the adult children who were living at home. She turned off the Internet at night so there was no access to online pornography. She required each person living in the house to take one chore. And she started charging rent.

It took a great deal of courage for Jeanette to enter into therapy with her children and listen to the stories they told. She learned it was okay to say no and to set limits, despite the guilt she felt about their childhood trauma. After slowly understanding how her sexual abuse molded her behavior and relationships, how her abuse set the stage for her children's maltreatment, she stepped away from the role of a fourteen-year-old whose sexuality was awakened too early—a teen trapped by a molester—and walked into her life as an adult who could receive love from others.

The blinders that she unknowingly wore from her trauma, and which put her children at risk for sexual trauma, had been removed once and for all. With continued hard work, her children and her grandchildren could live safer lives.

ALEX

How do I love thee? Let me count the ways.
I love thee to the depth and breadth and height
My soul can reach, when feeling out of sight
For the ends of Being and ideal grace.
I love thee to the level of every day's
Most quiet need, by sun and candle-light.
I love thee freely, as men strive for right.
I love thee purely, as they turn from praise.
I love thee with the passion put to use
In my old griefs, and with my childhood's faith.
I love thee with a love I seemed to lose
With my lost saints. I love thee with the breath,
Smiles, tears, of all my life; and, if God choose,
I shall but love thee better after death.
—Elizabeth Barret Browning

THE SUMMER AFTER MY FIRST YEAR IN GRADUATE SCHOOL, I moved to New York City and lived with Emily, a good friend. We shared a one-bedroom apartment on 92nd and Broadway. Upon returning to the apartment after my first day on Wall Street as a temporary secretary, I could not unlock the door. There were three deadbolts, and I was unlocking one and locking two, unlocking two and locking one.

Panic hit when a voice behind me said, "Do you need help?"

In exasperation and fear, I turned around and said, "Yes."

Dressed in a three-piece suit and holding the keys to his apartment, he looked harmless. Obviously, he lived in the building, and it appeared I was locked out forever, so I handed him the keys. After quietly unlocking the door, he gave me back the keys and walked away.

"Hey, Emily," I said, when she got home hours later, "a cute guy lives upstairs. He might interest you, but boy is he rude. He helped me into the apartment, then didn't even introduce himself."

"Why would I want to date a rude guy, Julia? Thanks, but no thanks. You can have him."

Alex, the man who opened my door, had a dramatically different reaction.

"I've met the girl I'm going to marry," he told his college roommate, later that week.

"What's her name?"

"I have no idea, but I'm going to find out."

Find out, he did. And after months of following me around and asking me out, we were a couple. We dated for one year, and although he knew he was going to marry me on the first day we met, determining the date was more problematic.

One night we were walking down Broadway and he told me rather rudely, that he "might rather own an old pickup truck, like that one, than be married." His final answer was no.

"How about an old truck and a wife?" I said.

To make things even more confusing, late that summer I got a phone call telling me I had been rejected from McMaster. Devastated, I decided to move back to North Carolina, where there were four medical schools and more physician spots per capita than in any other state in the country. I wanted one of them. But Alex was not convinced that changing jobs and moving to North Carolina was in his best interests. So I moved on my own.

I owe his dying cousin, Rod, gratitude for the gift of my life with him. At age twenty-seven, Rod was in Memorial Sloan Kettering Cancer Center, with malignant neuroblastoma. He suffered back pain for a year before it was diagnosed. Alex visited Rod in the hospital, eating the Ray's Pizza he had brought for the two of them, while Rod smoked pot that was prescribed to stimulate his appetite and decrease his nausea. Alex talked about me, and Rod listened with the ears of someone who would never marry, never have children, maybe never even leave the hospital. It was with Rod's encouragement that Alex started looking for jobs in North Carolina. He was moving, too—apartments 1F and 2J were merging.

Our November wedding filled Chestnut Street United Methodist to overflowing. I like to say that I got married and my mother invited five hundred of her closest friends, perhaps because it is true.

After moving down a few weeks before our wedding, Alex started working at Wachovia Bank in Winston-Salem, North Carolina. Applications to medical schools were submitted, and I enrolled at the University of North Carolina at Greensboro for my pre-med requirements. All I had to do was make high marks in physics, organic chemistry, and inorganic chemistry to gain acceptance to medical school.

MEDICAL SCHOOL

*I swear to fulfill, to the best of my ability
and judgment, this covenant:
I will respect the hard-won scientific gains
of those physicians in whose steps I walk,
and gladly share such knowledge as is mine
with those who are to follow.*
—Hippocratic Oath

OUR MEDICAL CLASS COMPRISED one hundred and three students, including thirty-four females, which was a lot for this small, private Baptist school in North Carolina—Bowman Gray Medical School, now known as Wake Forest Medical School. Although many of our female professors were unmarried, none of us considered choosing between family and medicine. We never considered the sacrifices we would make for *having it all*; never wondered about the cost to ourselves or to our families.

Since I had been active in an undergraduate women's association at UNC, I eagerly joined the American Medical Women's Association (AMWA). In second year, I was elected president. One morning, shortly after an AMWA fundraiser, I awoke to find our house had been egged. Fear and anger among the male students towards an organization that excluded men created animosity, and I lost several friends.

Gradually, the anger diminished, but a feminist label had been applied and it stuck. It didn't matter that I was friendly, happily married, and interested in relationships with both sexes. I had to live with my choice—leading a female organization and supporting women in medicine. After learning a valuable lesson about how quickly stereotypes and judgments are formed, I realized how difficult they are to change, and how much they hurt.

As the years of class work came to a close, the excitement and suspense regarding clinical rotations was contagious. With equal parts enthusiasm and naiveté, we marched into our patients' lives. Upon entering the hospital just as an epidemic of immunocompromised infections had erupted, we found patients dying of rare diseases that hadn't been seen in decades. Infectious Disease was working day and night to find the mechanism for an illness later defined as Acquired Immunodeficiency Syndrome (AIDS). Terror ran rampant throughout the hospital. Most of the students accepted the risks involved in practicing medicine, working in Intensive Care covered in masks and gowns, ministering to the sick. A few students refused.

That the illness primarily affected homosexual men was well-documented by that time, but no one knew the mode of transmission or that the virus lasted only hours outside bodily fluids. We did know that we didn't want to waste away while a fungus ate our lungs and skin. We knew we didn't want to die as we met the life-threatening consequences of our decision to become doctors.

AMBER

No murder.

—Exodus 20:13

A DEAD-ON-ARRIVAL CALL ALERTED US to Amber's entry into our ER, around midnight. Just three months old, she was actually unconscious, not dead. None of us had much experience with childhood neglect and abuse, but this patient provided a collision course.

"Epinephrine stat. Who's got the arterial line? Get that catheter in, pronto."

We were working against the clock, and fought hard, but there was no movement in her limbs, no light in her eyes, and she demonstrated no fear or pain during the many medical procedures. Her parents' reactions were also abnormal. There was no sense of injustice or sorrow as they were questioned. No life shone in anyone, baby or parents.

Many hours and procedures later, Amber was placed on a ventilator and transferred to the pediatric ICU. Based on Amber's physical findings, our attending physician in pediatrics called and reported the father for abuse. The father, the primary caregiver, was questioned.

Police reported that there were blood stains on the baby's changing table. Retinal hemorrhages, the hallmark of shaken baby syndrome, were present. He confessed to "being rough with her" before putting her down for a nap.

"When she slept for so long without waking for a bottle, I went and found her like this, not breathing," he said, in a dead monotone.

His flat, dispassionate voice made the hair on the back of my neck stand. This instinctual response became a trusted reflex, and I grew to rely on it over the years. But since this was my first brush with abuse in a medical setting, I was unsure.

Later, our attending told us, "The case is weak. Don't take sides or hope for the charges to stick. Don't get involved emotionally or discuss this with the family. Just take good care of Amber for as long as she is with us."

The police continued investigating despite how unusual it was for parents to be charged with the murder of their children at the time.

Our grief for Amber was palpable, so dense that it physically compressed us as we walked the halls of the Pediatric Intensive Care Unit (PICU). We knew from the first physical exam that Amber was not going to live, yet day after day she remained on the ventilator. Watching her slow decline was heartbreaking. After completing rounds, several students returned to her crib and bowed their heads in prayer over her little body, asking for a faster death and no pain, pleading for forgiveness as they witnessed a possible murder without consequences.

"We are disconnecting the ventilator this morning, after rounds," our attending said. "Who will be there?"

Most of us from the pediatric ER were standing by Amber, watching as the doctors signed off on her life, waiting as the ventilator, now separated from her tiny trachea, no longer moved her chest up and down. And we wondered, as she slowly stopped breathing, how our own lives were being transformed.

Her parents were not there, and I deliberated if that could be used as evidence in a court of law, including their lack of reaction in the ER, their flat expressions during the initial interview, Amber's protracted hospitalization, their absence while we disconnected her life support? It was clear that the evidence against them was mounting.

> *Entering the empty stillness*
> *of her emergency room cubicle,*
> *we pursued first aid and electrical stimulation*
> *to revive the beats that were not hers.*
>
> *She stopped breathing and exited her body,*
> *a little soul wearing diapers into heaven.*
>
> *Retinal hemorrhages gave him away,*
> *yet the father cried, too, at her funeral,*
> *having told all that a weakened blood vessel*
> *defective from birth was the murderer.*
>
> *They all wept,*
> *even the fetus growing in the mother's womb,*
> *waiting to be born into her sister's dead life.*

It was in the shadow of this darkness that I cried out for things to be different. How could God create a world where babies were murdered by parents, and no one was held responsible? Evil to me was getting caught speeding on the way to the beach, or hating my parents for not letting me go to a rock concert with my boyfriend. But murder—especially the murder of an infant by a parent—was beyond belief.

Nothing had prepared me for the helplessness and anger I felt when our attending told us the police had dropped the charges. The retinal hemorrhages had not been enough to indict the father, despite his admission of physical roughness. Incredulous that the mother was pregnant with her second child, and no involvement with social services was recommended, we despaired.

"Where are you, God, in this murder?" I said. "Show yourself, or you're culpable, too. What role should protective services play in the oversight of this unborn child?" I argued.

During this first brush with trauma, we were taught only to treat physical symptoms and ignore causes. Neither colleagues' reactions nor the attending's neutrality offered solace. How could the new sister or brother be safe if the father was to provide care while the mother worked?

Gradually, we turned to other duties. Some children were being treated for cancer. We were conducting a diagnostic evaluation in an infant with a genetic defect, Trisomy 21. Asthma tents and wheezing could be heard throughout the halls.

Months later, we gathered as students, interns, and residents, with attending physicians, for a scientific discussion of Amber's death. It was my turn to present, and I was sure that my turbulent emotions would interfere with the lecture. Pointing to my poster, I incorrectly identified the retinal hemorrhages as corneal hemorrhages. Despite the fact that I was visibly shaken, the attending criticized me, allowing no exploration of the cause of death or our feelings. Only physical details and diagrams were reviewed.

Here is lesson number one from Amber's death: Physical abuse of children does not exist. And if it does, it's not helpful to speak of it because there is nothing you can do. And if you do speak of abuse, do it only in a scientific manner. No feelings allowed.

RALPH AND JACK

*I prayed for this child,
and God gave me what I asked for.*
—1 Samuel 1:27-28

RALPH, A YOUNG FATHER STRICKEN SUDDENLY with leukemia, and I met on an internal medicine rotation. Lying in bed and wasting rapidly, he refused treatment or visits from medical staff. He was ready to die and asked me to help his wife waive off the multiple medical teams. The chief resident gave his permission, and with a nod from our attending physician, I used my spare moments directing people away from Ralph's room. Basically, I was on-call for cigarette and food breaks for the family, but being joined by a medical student gave credibility to their plan. They were grateful, and in the last few weeks of Ralph's life, we danced a choreographed routine, protecting and nurturing, bringing comfort.

"I'm coming." I dropped the phone into its cradle and grabbed my khaki skirt and pink oxford shirt lying conveniently on the floor by the bed.

I had been off the internal medicine rotation for a few weeks when his wife called.

"He wanted you here with us," she said.

Jumping up, I abandoned my thoughts of conception and babies, and dashed up the hill to the hospital. I raced to the elevator and stepped in for the ride to his grieving family, knowing they would open their arms to me, and me to them.

And that's when I felt it—a small, fluttering somersault stuck and held for just a second.

I placed my hand over my lower abdomen. "Well, hello, little fellow. We've been waiting for you for a long time."

Jack was born seven and a half months later.

THE MATCH

Three stars and the moon came out last night,
embracing, a sign of union.
A blue Chevy running bright as any Easter egg
skidded into the twilight and sank
into the future that banked our hearts.
Skipping stars bore a promise,
sliding paths whispered secrets,
yet no one knew out loud.
The fiddle tune heard in the feathers was played
by three stars shooting the moon.

—Julia W. Burns, MD

SHOOTING THE MOON TO OUR SLIDING PATHS, that's the assignment for fourth-year medical students. We were choosing specialties, and the last year of medical school required making decisions that would affect us for the rest of our lives.

"Hey, Julia, have you decided whether you are doing psychiatry or obstetrics?" said Lauren, my study buddy and friend, as we walked the short block to our houses.

She had just gotten married, and she and her husband, Bruce, rented a house beside ours. Linking arms, we sauntered down the hill from the hospital.

"I'm matching in psychiatry," she said, "because Bruce is determined to find an orthopedic surgery residency near

Chicago. I want to be near my parents so we can start our family. I want a sweet baby, like your Jack."

It's true, I was fortunate. If my days were filled with death and disease, my evenings and nights were filled with nursing and spit-up. As soon as I got home, Jack's sighs closed round my ears as I swept him onto my chest. There he stayed until the time came to separate, and I walked back up the hill to the hospital. Donning a white coat and a swinging stethoscope, I changed from mother into doctor each morning.

I was ecstatic when I learned I was pregnant—talk about *over the moon*—but kept it secret as long as I could. Rotating on surgery during second trimester was no time to reveal that condition. Serving in the surgical suite was tricky, as operating rooms were heated to prevent naked bodies on the steel tables from getting chilled. Our gowns, masks, gloves, and hats heated our bodies as well, and occasionally students passed out. Swooning before the fall gave nurses time to escort a wobbly student out of the surgery suite. I never did faint, but felt like I might, standing there counting backward from one hundred by threes, concentrating to stay upright.

Hours were long because we had to stay until the last surgeon was out of the operating room. Only after that could checkout rounds commence. That meant I might be finished at 5:45 p.m., but would be required to stay in the hospital until much later, when we gathered as a group to review patients.

After slipping out of the hospital early, I hurried home to put six-month-old Jack to bed, and rushed back before rounds. If you got caught, you were chastised or given extra work. An educated guess was required as to when the appendectomy in room six would finish.

Getting overheated in surgery happened in more than one way. Surgical residents were cocky and self-assured. They had little time for students except to make our lives miserable.

Once, as we entered the room of a woman who was recovering from a mastectomy, the chief resident on surgery joked, "Why did God give women two breasts? So we could take one."

I didn't say anything that day, but toward the end of my surgical rotation, it felt safer to challenge his behavior.

After another joke, I said, "I don't think that's funny."

The group of handsome, gifted men only laughed more loudly, ignoring me. But our patient looked up as we entered her room, and as the chief resident inspected the bandages covering her chest where her breast had lain yesterday, she said, "Yes, and I want you to know that I don't think it was funny either."

Then there was quiet.

By focusing on the good, I adapted. There were so many blessings. Jack cried, but he never yelled, and the flexibility of fourth-year was great for having an infant. We studied in the radiology lab together, examining X-rays, diagnosing fractures and pneumonia. We had lunch together every day, his nanny and I chatting as he nursed. And we rocked every evening on the front porch swing, listening for his father's footsteps as he walked up the sidewalk toward home.

Psychiatry appeared to be winning over obstetrics for my residency. Both would require a strenuous application process and then a wait-and-see period. Computers compared applications, and jobs were offered as students *matched* with schools. As toilsome as the process was for single students, it was particularly harrowing for couples because of the timing. Residencies were announced in mid-fall, but did not start until the next July. How was Alex going to keep our move a secret from Wachovia for nine months? It was going to be awkward.

Constructing a chart of the pros and cons of both specialties, I filled a notebook. Psychiatry got positive checks for schedule flexibility, reimbursement for time spent face-to-face with patients, and close relationships. OB-GYN's rigorous on-call schedule was a negative, but the primary care duties, combined with the surgical opportunities, were compelling.

The answer which had eluded me all year became certain during my labor with Jack. I'd been in labor off and on for fifteen hours, with no progress.

Dr. Meyers checked for cervical dilatation, and I said, "So, Dr. Meyers, am I in labor?"

He was embarrassed. I had been working on his research team for the past two years. We were friends as well as colleagues. I loved his wife's Mexican chicken casserole, something I really wanted now because they wouldn't let me eat. I wanted a precise answer.

I'll never forget what he said: "Well, Julia, labor is defined as uterine contractions with cervical change. It's not clear if that's the case here."

And I thought, *If these doctors and nurses, with all these machines and monitors, can't figure out whether or not I'm in labor, then it's obstetrics that's voodoo, not psychiatry.*

I doubt if Dr. Meyers had any idea how his answer affected my career, but my mind was made up. I began the process of completing psychiatry residency applications soon after Jack and I left the hospital.

100 STRAWBERRY STREET

Keep watch over me and keep me out of trouble;.
Don't let me down when I run to you.
Use all your skill to put me together. I want to see
your finished product.
—Psalm 25:20-21

"Alex, in five years I'll finish my training. You will be a senior officer at the bank, and Jack will be in first grade. Our hard work will come to fruition. Dreams do come true." I mused, changing another dirty diaper.

We renovated a downtown house in the historic district and couldn't imagine a better life than living in an urban area with art galleries, museums and concert venues, a tertiary care center, and a successful investment firm. Alex's job started immediately, so I finished fourth-year medical school remotely, taking electives which fulfilled all outstanding requirements. After graduating from medical school that May, I started residency in early July.

Manning the pediatric emergency room was interesting: a revolving door of crises laced with "sniffles for the past three weeks." Often, asthmatic children were brought by ambulance in the middle of the night. Sometimes their mothers disappeared before the children were stabilized with epinephrine and nebulizers.

"Julia, every room is full, and both nine and four are emergencies. Check with the triage nurse and make sure the waiting room is stable."

Infectious diseases, stitches, mental illness, asthma, abuse, and neglect—I saw all these on a single shift.

"Some mothers stop their children's medications so the hospital can provide daycare for three to five days," our chief resident explained.

I doubted her, but as I witnessed children returning frequently for the same symptoms—shortness of breath and wheezing—I wondered.

The neglect and abuse we saw in the E.R. made our jobs more difficult. At the time, I was grateful to assess physical diseases, leaving abuse to social services. It was their job to arrange follow-up, set up foster care placements and homeless shelters for patients in need. Evaluating adverse childhood experiences was not routine, and although we saw neglect and abuse, we consulted with social workers only rarely. Some scarring and burns were investigated, but seldom were children removed from their homes. Together, quietly supporting and teaching each other through our fatigue, we attended the medically sick, mostly ignoring the social problems.

Moving from a Baptist hospital in North Carolina to a more urban hospital in Virginia created challenges. The primary one came in the number of hours worked: thirty-six hours on, twenty-four off, thirty-six on. We worked in constant exhaustion during our six-week E.R. rotation. Heading for the resident's room, I'd lift up a quick plea that the emergency room would be empty from 2:00 a.m. to 5:00 a.m., but this rarely happened. There was little time for contemplation or prayer.

"How do you put a discharge address on the physical health form when the patient is homeless?" I said.

Frequently, 100 Strawberry Street would be the location given.

Finally, I asked the charge nurse, "How can so many families have the same address?"

"100 Strawberry Street is the homeless shelter, that's why" was the answer.

There were no moments to stop and reflect on how medicine was informing my faith. God had fashioned my path from childhood through college and early marriage, but recently I had paid little attention to him, going to church only occasionally, when it fit my busy schedule. My spiritual path meandered lazily through this physically exhausting year. I can't remember feeling his presence in the hospital, although I knew he could be found there. Instead, my energy was gathered into completing each duty and rushing home to be with Alex and Jack. They were always there, waiting for me.

As was God, if only I had noticed.

DON

Psyche means breath, spirit, soul.
Therapeia means healing.
Psychotherapy is soul healing.
—Anonymous

STORIES PILED UP IN EARNEST as I rotated through inpatient psychiatry wards and outpatient clinics: geriatrics, medical consultation, mood disorders, psychotic thought disorders, and addiction medicine. Patients were interested in talking, in giving an account of their lives. As I sat with them, my white coat pressed and buttoned, clipboard, pen, and paper ready, taking notes and listening, their words became a clinical summary that would open the door to healing. Carrying ten to twelve inpatients, I also evaluated one or two new admissions each day. Patients, especially psychiatric patients, can tell when you are distracted and rushed, and they don't like it. Staying grounded and present was imperative; they could easily tell a phony.

Once, I was physically threatened for casually giving a patient the news that his CAT scan was normal. He lunged at me with his fist cocked, pushed me against the wall, and threatened to punch me in the face because he was so frightened. He was having episodes of memory loss—finding himself far away from home, driving all night to another city. He was praying for a brain tumor over episodic fugue states, especially since his wife had recently died in her sleep from unknown causes. We all wondered if he had suffocated her.

After learning the valuable lesson that what is good news to the doctor may be bad news for the patient, I earnestly committed to discerning these subtle differences.

The outpatient clinic was next to the hospital, and all residents had to walk back and forth several times a day, scheduling individual and group sessions to fit other duties. Therapy cases were randomly assigned to residents by the director of the outpatient clinic, and each resident carried twelve patients. Picking up a patient who wanted to be seen twice weekly was good fortune, as it allowed in-depth examination of neuroses and behavioral patterns.

I was assigned one such patient: Don came on Tuesdays and Thursdays every week, for years. As I learned how to do psychotherapy, he gained insight into his self-defeating but life-saving personality traits. Sessions were taped for later review so they could be analyzed for content, inflection, and silent pauses. Dr. Weinstein, my clinical supervisor, and I met weekly for the meticulous but rewarding work, hunching over the tape recorder, listening to responses, discussing reactions, and assessing which explorations were helpful. Where should I have used silence or another intervention? When was I too quick to make an interpretation?

Don had a personality disorder that had been cultivated in early childhood. He remembered waking in fear, running through the halls, looking for a parent: "When I finally found someone, my parents would laugh at me, shaming and mocking me, and I trudged down the hall back to bed, dejected."

This happened often in his childhood, and he felt that the world was a hostile, uncaring place, and that he was unlovable. Much of our work centered around these themes, examining his frame of reference and supporting him. By encouraging him to find colleagues and friends who did not fit this paradigm, my consistent presence at 2:00 p.m. each Tuesday and Thursday was therapeutic. Because I never ridiculed or rejected him, no matter how many times he repeated the same angry accusations that I, too, was unloving and uncaring, we challenged his belief system.

"Hello, Don, come on in. We are in room five today. They had to move us because the air conditioner is broken in our room." Even a small adjustment like this would create dark moods and rigid withholding. Over time, Don was able to recognize that an air conditioner breaking was not my fault, but a mechanical failure that should not impede his progress.

We grew together. He gained awareness that his finger-pointing judgments rarely served him. I learned how to gently reflect this point.

After thirteen months of therapy, Don was able to ask women for dates and enjoy evenings with friends. His obsessions and compulsive checking behaviors—counting corners, cleaning and arranging objects—all decreased. He was promoted at work and was beginning to experience love.

JONATHAN

*There are wounds that never show on the body,
that are deeper and more hurtful
than anything that bleeds.*
—Laurell K. Hamilton

SEVEN-YEAR-OLD JONATHAN WALKED INTO THE OFFICE after his pediatrician referred him for "rule out autism." Lack of speech was the presenting problem, although Jonathan had spoken his first words at two years of age and continued to speak until the present. It wasn't autism that made him mute. It was trauma.

He was the oldest child in a drug-addicted family and was responsible for his younger siblings. If there was milk in the refrigerator, he filled bottles. He changed dirty diapers, if there were clean ones. Jonathan reluctantly went to school, leaving his younger siblings at home. A year ago, Jonathan's parents had gone to jail for drug trafficking, and the children's placement in foster care was mandated. Jonathan did not want to go to foster care, because his previous experience had been abusive.

His teacher reported that Jonathan attended school with welts on his legs. Jonathan was back home, and his parents were using meth again. This time, he kept silent because he didn't want trouble. Social Services had investigated multiple times after calls from the grandmother, teachers, and neighbors. Each time, the home was judged to be "safe," and the case was closed due to lack of evidence.

The parents, angry that they had been reported, barred the grandmother from seeing her grandchildren, cutting off all communication. Jonathan wanted to stay home, where his fate was known and he could keep his siblings safe. He did a good job, until one day his parents' drug use got so heavy that there was no milk or diapers. Still, Jonathan kept quiet.

When the telephone was working, his grandmother called the house, trying to assess safety. "Jonathan, how are you? How's Michael?"

Jonathan continually denied any trouble. Betrayal had come with too high a price before, so Jonathan protected the family. But he stopped talking the day the paramedics took his brother to the morgue and his parents to jail. This time, the charges were drug trafficking and murder. Jonathan and his remaining siblings were placed in the custody of his grandmother, and she struggled to care for them physically, emotionally, and financially. When Jonathan remained mute for six months, his grandmother saw a need for therapy.

He and I played together every Monday as he acted out his memories, smacking a baby on the bottom for crying, ignoring the doll in the crib. The dolls wrestled and fought until Dad looked over from his chair, jumped up, and spanked them. After locking the dolls in a closet, he slammed the door hard, and put the key in his pocket. While playing out many terrors and nightmares, he never spoke.

Who called the morgue when they discovered the baby with the dirty diaper, dead in his crib? I've never been told how long it takes a two-year-old to starve to death. Who cried out when they realized that the drugging and tripping took days? Who drove the maternal grandmother to the house to pick up the living children while the parents were fingerprinted and booked? Who cried for the baby at the graveside burial, and was Jonathan there? Who weeps now for the grandmother, custodian of five? Who grieves for the little boy who cannot speak, for if he does regain speech, will he tell of a brother who died in his crib, stench so deep that the paramedics had to cover their noses when they entered the room?

Speaking might have made a difference then, but how does a small child say the words that will betray his parents, save his little brother's life, and change his forever?

I never heard him speak, although I did bless him and his grandmother, praying for their safety and healing. And that's how I came to know Jonathan, who had nothing to say about his parent's drug use, or his little brother's whimpers of starvation— nothing to say ever after, either.

I tell you this story so you can witness our Mondays, sit on the floor with us, playing with therapy dolls in a dollhouse, listening to silent screams so loud we can all hear him now. Reverberations echoing down the hall, into the waiting room, where his grandmother sat watching four siblings, wondering if this would be the day when he opened his mouth and sound would come, or if silence would be his only language.

VETERANS

He holds in his hands our all, our life.
He holds in his hands our breath.
Breathing can be difficult sometimes,
and so remember this:
When you inhale, you taste him,
and when you exhale, he tastes you.
He holds in his hands our all, our life.
He holds in his hands each of you.
—Julia W. Burns, MD

IN OUR STRENUOUS THIRD YEAR, we psychiatry residents worked in the main civilian hospital and in the Veterans Affairs (VA) hospital and clinics. There, I encountered so much madness and despair that I questioned God again. Even though I knew he held me in his hands, I began to notice my own difficulties when I heard another story of suffering. It was in the face of this danger that my work with patients continued, and my relationship with God fell into distrust. Surprised by the trauma that greeted me every day, and disappointed by the higher power that allowed such chaos, instead of honoring God as creator of all—both health and suffering—I rebuked his wisdom and love. Rarely resting in his presence without accusation and questioning, I was hemmed in on all sides.

Since women seek therapy more routinely, it is unusual to see males for psychotherapy. Men typically wait until they are extremely ill before seeking intervention, so the pathology ran pure, distinct, and deep.

"Dr. Burns, it's cold in here," Robert said. "Do you hear the souls of the dead? I killed hundreds, thousands. I don't even know…so many I lost count. I went undercover at night, slipping into tents and slitting throats with my team. We stayed while they choked on their blood, making sure they were dead. Do you hear that, Dr. Burns? I hear it every day. Can you feel it? I'm freezing, always so cold."

"I feel it," was all I could say. Shivering, though it was summer.

We both felt death.

Robert and his wife had driven over one hundred fifty miles to the clinic. No longer able to go to the hospital where he worked as a janitor, he was desperate and suicidal, spending most of his time sitting by the river that ran through his farm, ready to jump into the rapids, his only thought escape. He had no desire to live, no hope of peace. His emptiness and agony were disturbing.

To help him survive, I prescribed antidepressants, which did little to curb the numbness and suicidal ideation. Attending group therapy, taking his medication, this soldier mourned the loss of his own life. The life that could have been, without the minefields and the slaughter.

As he stumbled over his memories years later, we discussed the panic, the bombs, the dead, the sleep that never came, the nightmares that did. What remains when you're crouching by the river, trembling with self-loathing and destruction, trying to remember your name?

And then there was Bill, a bipolar veteran, who asked daily, for weeks, "Doctor, can you comb these maggots out of my hair? It itches."

His scalp was red and bleeding from the scratching. One duty awaiting the nurses was to cut his fingernails in hopes that the scabs could heal.

As his delusion faded, he was able to participate in group and family therapy. Shame consumed him because he had wasted his family's savings on a foolish business venture. His wife was angry, but they were working on reclaiming their relationship and their lives. They established safeguards to prevent financial ruin if he became manic again. He seemed ready for discharge.

Two weeks after his discharge, Bill called. The desk clerk did not interrupt morning rounds to inform me of the phone call. Our attending physician frowned on disruptions during rounds. Later, when I called back, Bill didn't answer. The desk clerk noted that he had merely asked for me. But after he hung up, he shot himself. My first suicide.

He wasn't even my patient, although I had discharged him since I was covering for another doctor. I kept wishing I had a chance to do it over. Guilt consumed me, concern that I hadn't listened on the day he left the hospital when he kept asking for medication directions.

"Dr. Burns, can you come here? I need to know if I take the lithium, two tablets in the morning and two at night, or all at night. I used to take them in the morning, but I think the directions on this bottle say night. Is that correct?"

He kept asking me how to take what, when. I didn't hear the real question, so I kept giving him the same answer.

"Yes, Bill, take two tablets in the morning and two at night. Anything else?"

What I should have heard was, *Help me. I'm not ready for discharge. I think about death. I'm numb and afraid.*

The inpatient hospitalization had diminished the voices and the delusional thinking, but not his fear. So in desperation, he killed himself—making the sadness, the numbness, stop.

Suicide and suicidal threats are extreme self-destructive behaviors. Dark emotions sometimes carry a patient into the abyss, where you can't reach them. Walking into that black madness, but not being caught or swallowed by it, takes practice.

When Bill killed himself, I was four months pregnant with Benjamin, our second son, and wondered how it marked us. Whatever our emotions were, we felt them together. Benjamin means *son of my right side, or son of my pain.*

BARRY

*The paradox of trauma is that it has
both the power to destroy
and the power to transform and resurrect.*
—Peter Levine

CONSULTATIONS IN THE VA emergency room were frequent—we saw patients with bipolar disorder, psychotic features, mood disorders, post-traumatic stress disorder, and alcohol and drug addiction. My knowledge of war trauma grew, and I saw many veterans who were often intact physically, but unable to work or enjoy relationships because of mental anguish.

Barry, my new intensive patient, and I worked together for two years. He kept a journal of war atrocities. He told me about watching children evaporate when explosions hit. The vision haunted and broke him.

Barry's father and maternal grandfather were alcoholics. His mother, a strong and dominating force in his life, demanded that he attend church on Sunday with his family. He met her with stubborn resistance as his emotional numbness and need for isolation challenged the intimacy required from his family.

He was angry, seething. When he spoke, even though his voice was soft, he smoldered. Abandonment, his main therapeutic and developmental issue, was relived as he told story after story about growing up as the oldest child of a single mother who had to work long hours to feed the family. He did not know his father, although his maternal grandfather was involved with the family. This grandfather drank, often using the family's limited resources for alcohol. He recalled his grandfather demanding that Barry purchase liquor, even as he lay dying of liver disease. Barry had trouble setting boundaries and saying no. The rage he felt when his needs were violated was reviewed in therapy, repeatedly.

"I had to go to the liquor store that day. I had to walk there, leaving my younger brothers and sisters alone. Ma was at work. I got back with the bourbon, and he drank it. He died later that day, still drunk. I killed him."

Smothered with shame, Barry could barely access words to describe his feelings. He could not see the scenario any differently, no matter how I reworded it to include that because he was a child, he could not be guilty.

His stories of Vietnam were also of loss and abandonment: "I was traveling in a convoy over remote hills, and got a flat tire. The soldiers in my troop laughed and left me to change the tire alone. I wandered aimlessly, attempting to find my way back to camp, without directions. I finally made it back because I ran into another convoy and they guided me to base."

These episodes of betrayal in Vietnam were frequent for Barry. Stories of being wounded and without shelter, frightened in villages without transportation, filled his journal. Marijuana and heroin were "passed around like candy," and he was constantly high. He continued to struggle with addiction to marijuana, which increased his apathy, social isolation, paranoia, and disconnection, but eased his hyperarousal, hypervigilance, and insomnia.

Barry remembered only deprivation and betrayal from birth to the present. Every time his mother got pregnant, he had to assume more responsibility. As the oldest of six, he was seething when he learned what I could no longer keep secret, that I was pregnant. He became quiet and withholding. I knew he was hurting, even as I worked hard to fulfill the requirements of third year.

Our sessions continued. However, little was accomplished. Benjamin's delivery date was close, and when I left for maternity leave, Barry was transferred to another resident, a male this time.

When a child embraces daisy cutter bombs,
she holds her arms skyward,
reaching up and outward, trying to grasp
either blue or yellow air.

As bombs burst fire from their center,
this child evaporates and rains hell, too.

What bones are left to scatter on her grave?

Listen, because before this splintering,
a breath surges past her lips
as every word of life releases.

Hear this rushing, this whispering?

Suddenly, wasted love and fear are flying free.

This happens before the splintering,

before all language is lost in ether,

and only then can her body evaporate as spirit
releases in the showering fire.

And you know, there was one last effort to heal,

before she gave way to wonder.

BENJAMIN

The right hand is God's special space—the place of honor. And because you are "son" of the right hand, that means you will grow up into that special space.
—Hebrew saying

ALTHOUGH I LEARNED MUCH, my third year was difficult. I underestimated the demands of the commute to the VA hospital, the depth of the soldiers' wounds. I was managing gestational diabetes again, and was glad when Benjamin was born. As much as I appreciated the training, I was ready to escape the stories of war and the strain of pregnancy. Fortunately, Benjamin was tough, too, and together we made it.

Two months after Jack celebrated his third birthday with the Ninja Turtles, I was in labor.

"Good thing Julia is a doctor, or there wouldn't have been one at Benjamin's birth," Alex said to whoever would listen. When he got the bill, I heard him mutter, "I wonder how much they charge when the doctor actually shows up."

I was grateful. Benjamin was so ready for his life with us that I only labored twenty minutes, and that is the perfect amount of time to lie on a labor bed. Benjamin slipped out between the sheets as they were transferring me to the high-risk delivery suite—all by himself. They ignored me when I said, "The baby is coming!" But after all the excitement, it was love at first sight.

Benjamin was so beautiful. His blond, wispy hair and his cherubic, round face stole our hearts. My most beautiful baby, as well as the most demanding. He nursed like a fiend, for months. I can't remember doing much else that summer except occasionally handing him off to Alex to play with Jack or grab a quick nap.

When October came, my thoughts turned again to psychiatry and the transition from nursing babies to treating patients. Pumping milk in the bathroom stalls was a skill I quickly acquired because Benjamin refused a bottle from me and everything but bottled breast milk from others.

I cried more than my children that year. Driving up the hill to the hospital, I missed them so. Of course, I thought about taking more time off, but decided it was better to stay on track and finish my training on schedule. I was going to be thirty-five when I completed my fellowship and wanted to graduate and look for a part-time job so I could be home with the children.

Pleading with God to capture my grief and usher me back into the world of psychiatry, I pondered the future. Would I continue to minister to veterans, or turn my attention to the college students that were attending the new group I was forming at the local university? I struggled and had difficulty concentrating. Not trusting myself, but not wanting to ask others for their advice either, I felt trapped.

Luckily, Benjamin was equipped, able to fight off the bad guys, even as his mother strained. He was our courageous warrior, trailing long chains of toy swords as soon as he could walk. He triumphed everywhere. After starting school, those plastic weapons became mystical and invisible, but he continued to carry them, surrounding himself with their power.

"On guard! Prepare to eat thy doom," he said to everyone he encountered.

The addition of Benjamin to our family increased the mayhem and the love, and we depended greatly on our sitter, Mary. Jack enjoyed putting puzzles together with her as she swaddled Benjamin in her large bosom. Many days, as I left for work, I envied Mary's position.

CHILD FELLOWSHIP

The parent-child connection is the most powerful mental health intervention known to mankind.
—Bessel van der Kolk

TWO BABIES AND THREE YEARS IN ADULT PSYCHIATRY brought me to the children's treatment center for my fellowship. The trauma stories I heard at the VA were merely a warmup for the stories I was going to hear from my pediatric cases.

A typical workday was eight to five, Monday through Friday. We took turns on-call for emergencies, one weekend each month. As the physical demands lessened, I had more time for reflection, and a more manageable work schedule allowed my relationships with friends and family to flourish. We joined a downtown Episcopal church and attended weekly. I taught Jack's three-year-old Sunday School class, enamored with the natural inquisitiveness and faith my students held.

Juggling the demands of our growing family took a toll. But that August, our extended family came together in a magnificent celebration—Benjamin's christening. He wore the long white gown that his brother wore three years earlier. Momma and her sisters came with sweet tea, vinegar pork barbecue, homemade rolls, Brunswick stew, slaw, and corn sticks. There were seven desserts, including Momma's famous pound cake. A harpist played while the children danced around the foyer. Alex purchased a keg of beer to go with the sweet tea—our cultural heritages, Scotch-Irish and Eastern North Carolina, combining to create new family traditions.

Jack played with his cousins in a big plastic jungle gym, sliding and climbing. Benjamin, with his round face and joyful smile, was passed around that day like a package, yet retained his sweet disposition. The difficulties of managing our family around the lives of an investment banker and a doctor-in-training were shelved as we honored Benjamin's baptism and our commitment to God. That commitment felt right and led me to believe that I was placed in the Charlottesville community to grow with my family and to heal others.

A few months after the christening, we returned home and had to scare away robbers who were prying the kitchen window open. A few weeks later, Alex's 1966 Dodge Monaco was stolen while parked in front of our house. Then one afternoon, an emergency room patient stuck his head over the white picket fence in our backyard—while I was playing with Jack and Benjamin in their baby pool. These events kindled a desire to move, but finding time to look for houses proved problematic. Alex and I often saw houses separately, and ruled out some so the other didn't have to waste time.

"Cathy," I said to our new sitter, "you know I have to see my patients before the attending comes in at nine. You've got to be on time for work."

But she rarely was. Our tardy sitter, our house hunt, and the used red Peugeot wagon, which kept breaking down, all needed attention. I managed these things mostly on my own as Alex traveled. Much of our family time that fall was spent driving across Charlottesville to the car dealership for repairs, the children and I singing, "I like to eat, eat, eat apples and bananas," when what I really wanted to eat was the salesman who had sold me a lemon.

It was time for a new sitter, a new house, and a new car. I pored over applications from the nanny service, intent on solving one of our problems. Finally, I selected a young girl and interviewed her over the phone. The agency had vetted and bonded her, and she was on her way. Lisa graced our lives for the next year, giving calm, loving attention to the boys. We traded the sitter, the car, and bought a brick rancher—one that came with lots of children and bike paths, but no patients lurking behind fences in this graceful, old neighborhood.

IGNORANCE

One major obstacle is that society, as well as psychology and psychiatry, are not eager to invest in the prevention, education, and treatment of chronic traumatization and dissociation.
—Ellert R. S. Nijenhuis

"Sexual abuse affects one in four children, Alex. Twenty-eight percent of children are physically abused. Four to seven children die from maltreatment each day." I was stunned as I read from the journal article that Dr. Sadler, the director of the children's psychiatric hospital, had assigned.

How had I chosen child psychiatry without knowing this? Hard to imagine, but easier to explain. I never had a professor teach best practices for chronic PTSD in children; no lectures or journal articles delineated treatment.

Chronic PTSD symptoms are well-known in both children and adults now, but at the time, the DSM had no nomenclature for chronic pediatric trauma and no discussion of domestic violence, despite its epidemic proportions. Physical abuse was rarely discussed, and sexual abuse was not mentioned except as an afterthought, or what we called a "V code," aSupplementary Classification of Factors Influencing Health Status and Contact with Health Services but not a primary diagnosis which is reimbursable

The revelations of how abuse played a role in my pediatric patients' mental illnesses continued throughout my fourth year. Late one afternoon, I was evaluating an eight-year-old boy. He was hyperactive, hypersexual, and aggressive. Admission to the hospital was required to stabilize both his medications and mood swings which made him violent at home and at school. The boy's grandfather and mother brought the child to the hospital and were waiting for me to admit him. During the admission interview, there were subtle and repetitive clues that this might be a case of incest. The mother reported being the victim of multiple sexual assaults. The child's symptoms—aggression and sexual acting out—were consistent with sexual trauma. An eight-year-old should not know about intercourse or oral stimulation of genitalia. This child knew about both.

The next morning, during rounds, I tentatively broached the subject with Dr. Sadler, our attending. "It's possible that the grandfather is the father.

While I was interviewing the mother, the grandfather interrupted and persisted in dominating and obfuscating, especially when sexual trauma was reviewed. He and the mother were contradicting each other, and she refused to answer questions about the father's biological history."

"What proof do you have of incest, Dr. Burns?" said Dr. Sadler.

"No confession, no proof, but the situation includes family secrets, contradictory history about the father, and sexual acting out in the boy. Also, the mother dissociates, and she endorses memory blocks. Almost half of children who are raped are victims of family members. Science backs me up."

But he dismissed the discussion, and I was taught to keep quiet. Incest and sexual abuse don't exist unless you can prove it. But denying and ignoring abuse impacted the care of our young patients. It may have also contributed to a tragedy on the inpatient unit.

A pediatric resident, Stewart, volunteered on weekends when nursing staff was low. One Saturday, a nurse saw Stewart engaged in sexual activity with a patient, and reported the incident to the clinical director. Later, she went to the police. The pediatric resident was charged with multiple counts of sodomy and assault of several minors. The trial lasted for months.

Our weekly conferences would have been a good time to explore the case against the young doctor and the trauma inflicted on the patients, but we only fleetingly discussed the case—long enough to learn that all the attending physicians believed the resident was innocent. I remember thinking that was doubtful. The nurse's eyewitness account, the victims' testimonies, and the number of charges filed by the state suggested otherwise.

The resident was found not guilty, finished pediatric training, married, and moved to Florida. Despite the faculty's assurance of his innocence, I continued to believe in his guilt. It seemed impossible that a nurse and these young boys would lie or makeup such specific details. I felt sure the doctor would continue to sexually abuse his patients, and that there was little the legal or medical profession would do to stop him.

"Hal," I said to the other child fellow, "I just don't understand how Stewart was found innocent. There were multiple counts of molestation and sodomy of a minor, for Pete's sake, an eyewitness account, and several victims' reports."

"Julia, don't you understand that if he had been found guilty, the hospital could have been held liable? The medical staff and the hospital could be ruined. Institutions resist disclosure because of culpability and liability."

"But what about the truth? What about all the victims he'll abuse in the future as a pediatrician?" I asked.

Hal nodded quietly. He knew about child molesters, because a priest in his village had been one. His friends who attended Catholic school shared stories: they had to take off their clothes and be weighed naked by the priest, one at a time, in the school bathroom while the nuns kept order outside the door. At the slightest misbehavior, the priest would smash his papal ring against their skull. Emotional, physical, and sexual assault were constant threats. As a result, several of his friends suffered from alcohol and drug addiction, living chaotic lives and dying early, some by suicide.

When Hal was five years old, he dared God to change his rubber knife into a real one so he could protect his friends. He felt impotent and angry when God failed to give him a steel knife and believed that he could not trust a God who turned his back on a little boy's prayers.

Much like Hal, as the doctor in charge of the adolescent unit, I found myself in the role of silent observer. Despite attending church regularly, I doubted and had no idea what to think or do about abuse, and no place, no God, to turn to for instruction.

Or at least, that's how I felt.

FRANK

*Trauma is not what happens to us,
but what we hold inside
in the absence of an empathetic witness.*
—Peter Levine

DISCOVERING THE EXTENSIVENESS of sexual molestation in my patients made me rethink an adolescent experience. A friend and I were in the local production of *Oklahoma* and rode to practice together.

"Hey Matthew, want a ride to play practice tonight? I might have to leave early. I have a Latin test tomorrow."

Matthew was unconventional, effeminate, and exceptionally intelligent. I was one of his few friends. We shared a love of learning and theatre. He was a genius in Latin, offering tutoring in exchange for rides.

That night, one of the adult male leads, Frank, said, "Go on home, Julia. I'll give Matt a ride."

Matthew called in tears the next day. "Luckily, I was able to fight him off."

We vowed to get revenge, and I never left Matthew at play practice again. A few Sundays later, my family sat in the pew behind Frank. A friend of my parents', a member of the church leadership team, and president of a large textile company, Frank wielded significant power in Robeson County. I squirmed through the service. Telling my parents that afternoon the story Matthew had told me was difficult, but I wanted Frank to get in trouble, arrested, or at least have our pastor informed.

Their response: "Julia, I'm sorry, but no harm was done. Matthew wasn't hurt. It's best to leave it alone."

Deeply troubled by their refusal to take Matthew's attempted rape seriously, I ran to my room, crying. I wanted Matthew to come over and convince them, but he said no. Everyone wanted the incident to be forgotten. If I had known then what I know now about the hundreds of children raped by a single perpetrator, I would have done more than cry. But I was only fifteen, and believed my parents were wise and knew that they were powerful.

Forty years later, I learned that Frank had been arrested and had served time for lewd sexual behavior. It did nothing to ease the memory of those painful, dark days when I was Matthew's only confidante.

RESEARCH ASSISTANT

*And it came to pass, when they brought them
forth abroad, that he said, Escape for thy life;
look not behind thee, neither stay thou
in all the plain; escape to the mountain,
lest thou be consumed.*

—Genesis 19:17

"Fuck you, Dr. Burns. I'm not taking your medicine," I might hear from a patient. After all, I was just another adult, one with power over their lives, one that might hurt them, too. Why should they trust me when the other authority figures in their life had been so untrustworthy?

I loved the honesty my pediatric and teen patients exhibited. Although compliance is often a problem with both young and old, younger patients don't obfuscate. An adult patient might come for months, complaining about depression, and answer questions about medication side effects, all the while the prescription is lying on the kitchen counter, unfilled.

Stories of abuse were unrelenting as my patients and I sat together. God's answers, never sufficient. My medicines, rarely enough. Others saw the abuse infrequently, but as I persevered, I inhabited my patients' lives and had no trouble believing them.

One spring day, I walked across the street from the Children's Treatment Center to explore the Department of Genetics. I met the primary investigator on a twin study researching the epidemiology of childhood mental illness. The department of child psychiatry had been excluded from their proposal to the National Institute of Health. My involvement would change this.

Dr. Sadler, my training director, was excited about the opportunity: "By all means, Julia, go and find out. If they will hire you, we can spare you one or two half-days a week. Remember, I'll consider it a failure if you graduate and see patients individually. The shortage of child psychiatrists is so dire that, ideally, you should work as a researcher, or with a team of professionals. Research will create opportunities for you to impact hundreds or thousands of lives, not just individuals. Multi-modal team approaches to treatment will maximize your ability to influence a larger population of patients."

After a brief interview, I was hired. I sat many hours at the computer, inputting data from raw numbers. Hidden behind the lens of researcher, and protected from the stories of my pediatric patients, I prayed, "Keep me here, Lord. This is where I belong."

After weighing Dr. Sadler's words, I completed my fellowship and prepared my resume: physician in charge of the children's unit and adolescent unit, consultation-liaison doctor—evaluating inpatients when their physical illnesses were influenced by psychiatric disorders. And now, I added *research assistant* to my resume.

GRAY

*For we think back through our mothers
if we are women.*
—Virginia Woolf

"Really, Julia, are you sure that having another child is a good idea? The boys are independent, and Benjamin is out of diapers. We just put the crib and changing table in the attic. Do you truly want to start over?"

Yes, I wanted to start over. A daughter, maybe two, was my desire. Soon, this wish became reality. The pregnancy in the last year of my fellowship was similar to the previous two. I had gestational diabetes and pre-term labor. But it was expected, and the schedule allowed more flexibility. I felt healthy.

One night, in my second trimester, we were sitting by the fire after the children were in bed, when a phone call came.

"We are looking to hire a president for our money management company," said a friend from Alex's small New England hometown of New Hampshire. "Do you know anyone?"

I wanted to stay in Virginia, near an academic institution, and continue research.

"I can't be that far from home," I said. "I'll miss everyone. And the weather! I don't want to do this."

"But it doesn't snow much anymore, " Alex replied. "And my mother will help with the children."

"But we already have my mother for that." I sensed my defeat, even as I argued.

In the end, we both had a vote. But as they say, *the one carried.* Agreeing that it was important to have our family together every night, I knew that wasn't possible if Alex continued in investment banking. The decision to take this job offer and move to his hometown was made. It was a sad time—finishing training, managing the last months of my pregnancy, preparing the house to be sold, and saying goodbye to friends and colleagues.

All unhappiness lifted when Gray arrived. She was everything I'd dreamed of. And if God can give you more than you can ask for or imagine, it was true with her. I went into labor on a sultry day, after entertaining thirteen three-year-olds at the pool, celebrating Benjamin's third birthday. It was a fun day of balloons, sticky fingers, soaking wet bottoms, and little mouths begging for corn dogs and another piece of ice cream cake. Later that evening, Momma and I were sitting under the carport, watching the boys on the swing set, when my water broke.

"Oh, no," I said.

I took terbutaline to stop pre-term labor, and I was afraid it might slow down the birth. My concern was well-placed, because Gray took her time; it was hours before we met. But then her love spilled over us, pouring out joy. She was a lovely distraction from the pain associated with the move, even if her birth did make it more complicated.

NEW HAMPSHIRE

*When I am dust to dust, my songs and stories
you won't sell. So listen and be kind...
I am about to burst with song.*
—Psalm 30:10

THE WAVERING RHYTHM WE SO TENUOUSLY established was disrupted by our move. Alex moved first, and when Gray was three months old, Jack, Benjamin, Gray, and I joined him in a rental house off the university's golf course. I had everything I wanted: three beautiful children, a medical degree with specialized training in adolescent and child psychiatry, a kind husband, and multiple job prospects. Yet I was devastated. Never dreaming that I'd hang my shingle in a rural setting, I missed my research and professional community, my family and my friends. Memories of the North Carolina beaches, where I spent much time in my childhood, floated through my mind, juxtaposed with an Auden poem, as I sat on the porch of our rental, rocking Gray, nursing and weeping.

*The ocean's waves called me home,
beckoning seductively.*

*How did it come to pass
that the rhythmic repetition
framing those beloved shores let me go?*

Did the seagulls put on crepe paper bows,
crooning goodbye as I departed?

Remember that sweet, solemn lament they sang,
woven in sorrowful notes?

Listen as that wailing sound drains the ocean
and puts out the stars until not even the moon
can lighten the night.

When did the hourglass fall,
sand dripping backward?

When did our old living pass?

Come back, come back. Please don't go.

Do you hear her drowning, the serpent asked,
early one morning at dawn?[8]

I didn't think to ask God what he thought, if his plans included a small village and a rural child welfare agency. I didn't care much about God or his plans, either way. I was too consumed with regret and despair.

Enduring week after week of rain our first summer up north, I was overwhelmed and exhausted from caring for three small children, especially as the weather kept us indoors. Lonely and homesick, I was looking for a job by the time Gray turned five months old.

In the summer, sometimes the rains come
and continue for so many days
that the furrows drown into moats,
so that even the earthworms float belly side up
and the skylark's song melts away.
The orange red blaze of the square-stemmed
bee balm hugs the mud until bees go hungry, too.

SONGS FOR THE FORGOTTEN

*As damp days plow on, some strangeness
  locks itself inside our chest.*

*Seduce us back into the land of the living,
  bring out the music and light the sun.*

*Listen for the harmonies, because the song sings
  once the rain stops.*

WHITE PINES

There can be no keener revelation of a society's soul than the way in which it treats its children. Let us reach out to the children. Let us do whatever we can to support their fight to rise above their pain and suffering.
—Nelson Mandela

WHILE INTERVIEWING AT WHITE PINES, a three-hundred-child welfare agency that specialized in a collaborative treatment-team approach, I met several childcare staff and residents. The executive director called within days; I was hired.

I had already started a part-time private practice, and given the lack of child psychiatrists, it wasn't long before I had a waiting list. Tourette's was a common diagnosis, and I saw more patients with tics in a few months than I thought I'd see in a lifetime. I called my old training director for supervision. We assessed verbal and motor tics and discussed medication efficacy.

Treating patients in residential care during that initial week remains etched in my mind. My only request was an office with a window. I understood early that my work required ventilation; stories of abuse needed to blow in and out. Regrettably, no windows were available, so concrete block walls in a basement office encased me. Two nurses, Joan and

Glenda, worked across the hall. They scheduled new patient appointments and medication follow-ups.

Residents' discharge planning started on the day of admission. The goal was their return home within six months. Monitoring abuse, mistreatment, and neglect was a priority as we assessed strengths and resources. At first, I couldn't understand why birth homes should be favored. But gradually, I recognized that with support and coaching, therapy and medication, many children were safe with their birth families. While the obstacles for returning home were steep, fostering a child had a different set of obstacles. Most parents *wanted* to care for their children, but poverty and their own abuse or addictions caused them to be neglectful and sometimes abusive.

My pediatric patients were ready to sing, and as the notes rang out, it took concentration to remain calm and focused. Even as I believed, I was incredulous. Remember, this was happening to a young psychiatrist who had received no training in childhood trauma, and had no idea how to process stories or how to protect myself after I heard them.

We took care of each other in our child fellowship when a therapist had a particularly difficult session with a patient. They would seek another provider to tell the story to, or asked for help processing a disturbing incident. I had a vague idea that the work I was doing could hurt, and that self-care was important, but no real direction about exactly how to do it.

Following the usual pattern with psychiatric evaluations, I started with the history of present illness. The presenting symptoms might be verbal and physical aggression, or sexual acting out and truancy, but the precursor to the disordered behaviors was abuse. Single mothers on crack neglected their babies and put six-year-olds in charge. Family members beat their children and began sexually grooming them in infancy. Children grew to react to trauma in the only language they spoke—fear and anger—which typically resulted in aggression.

Their violent behavior got them admitted to White Pines for six to eighteen months, and the child's aggression had to be modified for the family to be reunited. Assessing for the safety of each home, and teaching parents how to care for their children, was our job.

Reading everything I could on physical and sexual abuse, I scoured books and journals after my children went to bed. But the best instructors were my patients. They told me everything that had happened to them—at least, everything they could remember. Talking freely about their lives, they trusted me. Even though the DSM provided no schemata for the symptoms I was treating, it didn't take long to realize that five milligrams of Ritalin would not offer a cure. Stimulants were great for attention and concentration problems, but did not fully treat the hyperactivity, inattention, impulsivity, and aggression associated with chronic trauma or exposure to drugs in utero.

"Dr. Burns, I did not throw that chair at my teacher!" Joe said.

"Well, Joe, I'm having trouble with your story because the teacher says you did, and your classmates saw you, too."

Joe was ten years old, and we had been meeting monthly, for six months. He seemed sincere in his denial, and had never lied to me. It was puzzling. How could he invest in his treatment plan if he could not remember what he did, and did not think he had done it? Stimulant medication had improved his attention-deficit/hyperactivity disorder. More medication was not likely to be helpful.

Although lack of training in trauma left me ill-prepared, it was the overall dismissal of trauma and its impact on behavior that confounded me. There was no platform for the conversation, therefore it did not impact treatment. Fortunately, I was heading to New York City to the annual meeting of the Child and Adolescent Psychiatry Association. I had been appointed a founding member of the Child Abuse and Neglect Committee.

How is it that the American Academy of Child and Adolescent Psychiatry didn't found a committee on abuse and neglect until 1992?

MARILYN

*She was a stranger in her own life,
a tourist in her own body.*
—Melissa de la Cruz

ANXIOUS TO LEAVE WHITE PINES for the conference, I had high expectations that a mentor could assist me. I was looking forward to working with the founder of a family therapy institute that specialized in trauma and dissociation. Dr. Thomas and I met at the first meeting, and I asked for a consultation. Our meeting started with the complex case of a nine-year-old girl, Marilyn, who had been referred for residential treatment because of sexual acting out and aggression.

During her psychiatric evaluation, Marilyn had drawn eight pictures of herself, effectively giving a visual representation of her multiple personalities. One was an elegant, well-dressed woman, another a werewolf, another looked like Cinderella with a broom and dustpan...the characters of her life continued in detail.

When I asked her who the people in her drawings were, she calmly said, "I'm not sure." She then explained that the elegant lady was "good at sex." The girl in rags was "good at cleaning. The werewolf comes and protects me when mean men hurt my mom and me." There were others, but she didn't know them as well.

I knew of no mental illness consistent with the symptoms this young girl was presenting. Having been taught that multiple personality disorder was rarer than schizophrenia—less than 1 percent—I had no idea how often I would see multiples and dissociation in my first year of work. After suggesting to Dr. Thomas that perhaps this little girl was psychotic, I asked if she needed a major tranquilizer.

"What?" Dr. Thomas paced around the small conference room table. "If you do that, she will be misdiagnosed and mistreated by physicians for the rest of her life. No, you call her multiple personality disorder, because that's what she is."

"But how do you treat that?" I said.

He sighed. "The best chance she has is to leave her abusers and live in safety. Over time, she may be able to integrate her multiple selves. Hopefully, she can learn to trust others in non-abusive relationships. Unfortunately, sometimes traumatized children recreate violent relationships and abandonment because it feels familiar. For now, it is critical to manage her symptoms—aggression, inattention, insomnia, and hyperarousal—with medication. Behavioral and educational therapy will be integral in helping her stabilize her rage. Misdiagnosing will not help; it only sets patients up for ineffective treatment through the medical system, because anti-psychotics may curb the aggression, but will not treat the primary disorder. These children are not psychotic. They dissociate, separating parts of themselves so they do not go crazy. It's the abuse they are experiencing that is insane, and so they split it off from their consciousness. It makes no sense to them that the father who feeds them is the father who beats them and has sex with them. Separate parts attend to each demand, allowing them to function. They cannot integrate these abusive experiences. Dissociation is the only way they can live within the family."

As our consultation ended, I made a promise to Dr. Thomas: "That makes sense. I'll never diagnose a traumatized, dissociative child with schizophrenia. I promise."

When I returned to the agency, Marilyn and I wrote this story:

Once, there was a little girl who was good, but the adults she lived with hurt and scared her. Her father would go into rages and beat everyone in the family—the girl, her brother, and her mother. He also came into her room at night and forced her to do things that frightened her, things she did not understand, things that hurt her. The little girl never knew when this would happen or what to do to make it stop. She was so frightened when her father was in her room that she pretended she wasn't there. Since she couldn't walk out with her feet, she walked away in her mind. Imagining leaving the bedroom, she went outside to play. Any place was better than the bedroom with her father.

The girl tried to tell her mother, but her mother slapped her and told her not to lie, so the little girl had no place to go but inside her mind. Since she was safe there, she went more often, spending so much time in her imagination that it got harder to tell where she was, when, and what she had done. She separated her imagined selves into special talents: math, sex, cleaning, memorizing scripture; each one had a different expertise. Gradually, there was less communication between each self, and more memory lapses. Determined to keep the family secrets, the little girl concentrated hard, but soon things began to fall apart. The girl who was good at sex started going to school. Classmates told on her for asking them to do funny things on the playground or bathroom. She became more isolated and afraid.

A social worker came to her school to interview her. The little girl never told any secrets, but still she was referred and admitted to White Pines. This is when she started understanding and telling.

Marilyn looked up quietly, staring into my eyes as I read out loud, and said, "I know that girl. I told you that story because it's me."

In that moment, we both knew truth. Now it began to make sense. Neither of us knew how to protect her from her personalities, her beatings, her premature lessons in sodomy and oral sex. But she knew that I believed her. She knew I understood what had happened to her. We learned that dissociation and flashbacks made the trauma seem real, even though she was far away from her perpetrators.

Many years later, Marilyn was enrolled in classes at the local community college. She saw an advertisement for my workshop, *Moving Through Your Life Stories with Writing and Yoga,* and attended. In the workshop, participants journal about life experiences, then move into gentle stretching and yoga positions, attempting to move the stories out of the deep muscle tissues. Moving major muscle groups and releasing neurological patterns creates healing as the experiences stored in the emotional center, the amygdala, are rewritten and moved into the hippocampus, where it becomes narrative, not terror.

Marilyn was working hard to create a childhood for her daughter that she would not need to heal from.

DANGEROUS DARKNESS

But it took him a while to notice that while the mental health of his patients largely improved with each passing therapy session, his own was deteriorating.

—Aaron Reuben

THERE WAS NO TURNING BACK, because once you know something, it is impossible to not know it. As soon as I learned that trauma was the primary factor in a resident's behavioral problems, I had to take a history and include that history of physical and sexual abuse in the initial psychiatric evaluations. And once I began asking, a torrent rained down. The children rarely hesitated.

"Did anyone ever beat you or burn you?" I said. "Do you ever touch a grownup's private parts, or have them ask you to touch theirs?"

"Yes, my mom burns me with her cigarette when I'm bad or she's mad," Lewis replied.

"And," I venture, into what is now well-known territory, "what do you do that's bad?"

"I forget to feed my brother, and sometimes I hit my brother when he doesn't listen."

"And then she burns you?"

"Yes, while I stand in the corner."

"How long do you stand in the corner?"

"Oh, usually for two or three TV shows. I missed *SpongeBob SquarePants* on Friday, and that's my favorite."

Children measure time in TV shows. How can this be ignored as testimony for abuse? When can we refer this child to a foster family? What is happening to his siblings now that the scapegoat, or identified patient, Lewis, has been removed?

It was up to social services to review Lewis's case and make a recommendation for placement. Residents at White Pines were in a tiered system, with the highest functioning clients being referred to foster care. There were also therapeutic foster care homes, residential cottages, and detention. Now we were being asked to consider another treatment modality—a residential treatment facility (RTF)—which was one step below the level of care provided by the state hospital. New Hampshire had requested proposals for a RTF for emotionally disturbed adolescents and children.

White Pines was awarded the government contract, and proceeded with construction. It would have twelve beds for boys, six for girls, and would operate under the supervision of the Office of Mental Health (OMH). Three social workers, a team of nurses, a psychologist, a recreation therapist, a therapeutic cook, a clinical director, and a medical director would have oversight of the most aggressive and difficult to treat psychiatric patients in our area. The favorable staff-patient ratio—six patients to each therapist—would allow us to examine patients through the lens of trauma. Opportunities for staff trainings would be a priority, especially in-service classes about dissociation and post-traumatic stress disorder.

It was a great opportunity, and I was looking forward to the challenge, even though I would have to close the private practice I had worked hard to create.

Treatment at White Pines continued, typically addressing behavioral problems, such as verbal and physical aggression, with positive and negative reinforcement. Positive reinforcement included increased privileges, such as a later bedtime, or the opportunity to go off campus for field trips. Negative reinforcement might be loss of those privileges. The previous month, after much campaigning, punitive behavioral modifications, like standing in the corner, were no longer allowed. But while walking through the cottage one morning, I saw Albert, a thirteen-year-old resident, with his nose in the corner.

"Albert, what's going on?" I said.

"I don't know, Dr. Burns. I guess I forgot to straighten my room this morning. Then I mouthed off to Brian when he asked about it."

We had eliminated standing in the corner as a punishment. There had been some controversy over that decision, but compliance was mandatory once the leadership team's decision was made. Yet it appeared that some of our childcare staff were continuing to place children in the corner, forcing them to stand with their noses to the wall, replicating the abuse they received at home.

Albert's history—gleaned over many appointments—revealed more than ADHD. He had a long-standing physically abusive relationship with his mother. His treatment team sessions often ended with Albert and his mother engaged in a long kiss on the lips, or a screaming match that made everyone in the room uncomfortable.

> *Stuck like glue to the patch of shaved wood*
> *in the corner of the living room,*
> *TV blasting out his favorite superhero's escape,*
> *Albert plotted her death.*
> *Stripped and stretched naked, as he often was,*
> *Albert fantasized her demise.*

> *When his lower limbs numbed,*
> *and his upper ones fell, his mother cracked him*
> *on the back with the buckle for lack of obedience.*
>
> *Wetting his pants, he had been standing,*
> *stuck in the corner, for five hours*
> *and seventeen minutes when it happened.*
>
> *They united against him*
> *when she asked his brother to set the kettle,*
> *to purify the sin of the elder.*
>
> *We met him after the "cleansing" left*
> *a burned upper body and a scarred, numb soul,*
> *arms forever unfeeling, and an allegiance*
> *to tell no one how the kettle got lit,*
> *to be poured over the sacrifice of the elder son,*
> *who disobeyed when he dropped his arms*
> *and pissed his pants*
> *while serving his penance in the corner.*

And here he was, serving penance in the corner again. I marched straight to the executive director's office, determined to take a stand against punishment, particularly abusive punishments.

"Matt, I just left Cottage A and found Albert standing in the corner."

Matt was alone in his office, and I walked in without an appointment. It was not something that was encouraged, but he could tell I wanted to be heard.

"Is this something unusual?" he replied. "Have you seen this before?"

"Yes, it has been our practice, but the leadership team voted against punishments last month—specifically, standing residents in the corner. I thought this was clear, yet staff are violating agency policy. It's upsetting because this punishment is outdated, and I was hopeful that at last we were done with it."

"I'll talk to Zachary and have him draft another memo asking staff to follow policy. We can't tolerate childcare workers taking discipline into their own hands. Thank you for bringing it to my attention, Julia."

I left the meeting, heartened. But the next week, I saw Albert standing in the corner again. Of course he felt comfortable; so much of his childhood was spent there that he felt safe and in control. But he was also enraged.

Was the behavioral model used in the residential cottages at White Pines a good fit for our trauma residents? While the children's abusive histories remained a constant, the therapeutic milieu's response to their suffering seemed inadequate, and even abusive.

Matt's response seemed unlikely to mandate change. Our children were neglected and abused by their parents, yet the treatment center and on-grounds school remained ambivalent about post-traumatic stress disorder and its symptoms: hypervigilance, hyperarousal, numbness, flashbacks, social isolation, and angry outbursts. The children's fuses were simply waiting to be lit so their rage could explode.

And I was stuck in the middle.

RESIDENTIAL TREATMENT FACILITY

*For the law was given through Moses;
grace and truth came through Jesus Christ.*
—John 1:7

"Dr. Burns, you do realize that you will have to assess patients every half-hour if they are in a physical restraint?" Madeline, the clinical director, said during one of our many RTF pre-opening discussions.

The OMH was adamant about reducing physical restraints because a recently completed study had found that the majority of injuries to staff and patients occur while using restraints.

"They are going to have a close eye on us since we are the new facility."

Physicians had to check blood pressure, pulse, and mental status on patients every thirty minutes during restraints. Any incident required a detailed report analyzing the minutes and hours before the event. Although this meant significantly more work for the medical director and staff, the mandate and the oversight monitoring compliance was welcomed. The underlying commitment to the least restrictive level of care required that physical restraints were used only as a last resort.

As the construction for the RTF continued, excitement about the new treatment model grew. Treatment plans would be based on a clinical understanding of trauma as well as behavior. Hiring was underway, and several applicants were being considered for the social worker positions. They were plum jobs because of the low patient-to-staff ratio, but most applicants did not realize the severity of the patients' illnesses. Few understood the level of violence they were about to encounter, nor did they realize the nature of the abuse that our patients had experienced.

While transitioning into these new responsibilities, I made plans to work full-time at White Pines. Praying frequently, I asked God for his blessings on the staff, the patients, the building, and me. The worse the stories got, the more I searched scripture for answers and reasons. Arising early in the morning to read the Bible, I searched for commandments directing adults to abstain from sex with children. Incest was an ancient and primal behavior, but I found little evidence that God had spoken against it. The few notations in the Old Testament left me wanting more.

Paul, in his letters, discussed chastity as a way of purifying the body to make space for the holy, but there wasn't a specific admonition against sex with children. Jesus should have preached against it—perhaps that would have satisfied.

A media fast was put in place to give the illusion of control. I couldn't watch the tragedy of the news and then go to work and listen, so I gave up reading about or watching news stories.

At cocktail parties with friends, I cited an article recently published by the American Psychological Association that a significant percent of Catholic priests were child molesters. Remember, this was in the early nineties, and quoting this study to my Catholic friends created a barrier between me and everyone else. They stared incredulously, and I grew accustomed to those stares. Determined that the looks would never be a deterrent, I wasn't going to stop telling, ever.

As my awareness grew, I leaned hard into that dangerous darkness. If I suffered with my patients, surely my work was making a difference. I had to remain at White Pines, changing both the residents' lives and the paradigm for treatment. As my anger grew and my trust in a benevolent God faltered, I became increasingly lonely, dropping out of my book club and refusing social invitations, staying home, feeling safe only with my family and co-workers.

Patients filled my ears with tales of their abusive relationships with family members, teachers and principals, priests and church staff. Often, perpetrators were accused by the victims, yet the relationships were allowed to continue.

My imagination painted an all too vivid picture and I protested, "Where are you, God, in this drama?"

I got no answer.

Or no answer that I would accept.

BLACK BOX

Black box sits in your family room,
full of poison and destruction.
Flip the switch, surge—turn on that bright light
with images of pain and violence.
Black box sits full of poison, waiting to sting.
Turn it off, turn it off or darkness reigns.
—Julia W. Burns, MD

MY SONGS ABOUT THE DANGERS OF TELEVISION and video games was not embraced by the boys. They loved to tell about the time I dropped the television on my toe, attempting to put it back in the closet. And they begged incessantly for a Nintendo® and PG-13 movies.

"Everyone else gets to, Mom. Most of my friends play on school days. How about just weekends for Nintendo?"

They never wearied of the battle, especially my warrior, Benjamin. He was particularly creative and challenging.

"Mom, can I have a bagel?"

"Of course." I toasted the bagel and spread butter and cream cheese on, as usual.

"Sam's mom won't let him have butter and cream cheese. But she lets him play video games. If I give up cream cheese, can I have a Nintendo?"

Alex and I continually said no, but they chafed against our decisions. Although usually supportive, this time Momma interfered. She was coming for Easter, and orchestrated a trade. My nephew was selling his Nintendo and a shoebox full of games for one hundred dollars. I believe he wanted to buy a new bike, and Momma knew that Benjamin and Jack wanted those video games. My worst fears were realized: once the video games were installed, Benjamin would do nothing else. He would get red and become agitated with full-scale tantrums when asked to stop and come to the table for supper or to do his homework.

I donated all the video games to the RTF after one week.

"Dr. Burns, if you won't let your children play video games, do you think we should allow our residents?"

"Well, Madeline, that's up to you. But if our residents can have a few minutes of forgetting, and a bit of fun with a video game, that's good. If the games increase tantrums and aggression, then we should take them away."

I didn't tell her that the tantrums had exponentially increased at my house.

The cold and cloudy weather was burying me alive. When it wasn't snowing, it was raining. March in North Carolina brought warm, sunny weather, dogwoods and azaleas dripping with sensuous life. March in New Hampshire brought snow and cold. Spring in New Hampshire was called "mud season." My parents visited only between May and October. No one would venture north during the winter.

"When is spring coming? We are still wearing down coats!" I cried, as snow piled up outside our bay window, covering the sills on Mother's Day.

Spring soccer and May birthdays enticed Momma to visit.

She often said, "Julia, don't tell me you are going to let the children play soccer in this rain." More of a demand than a question.

I replied, "If they didn't play in the rain, Momma, they'd never play."

Songs of our home life continued, and I often mourned the interruption of the Sabbath by soccer games.

> *The Lord is my rock. So then rock me, Lord.*
>
> *Like a baby, I come to you filled with doubts,*
> *fears, and confusion about life, love,*
> *and what encircles a joyful world,*
> *and you greet me always with*
> *your light-filled days.*
>
> *Sun rising yet again to renew us,*
> *clarify your vision of how our world should rotate*
> *on your axis.*
>
> *Rock me, world. Rock away*
> *this discontent, skulking, pouting misery*
> *as I lie in the grass and listen to parents*
> *yelling for their team to score the goal,*
> *their child to stay alert and play well;*
> *not rejoicing in the little legs*
> *that run so fast after the ball at all.*
>
> *Rock me, Lord, I need a jolt,*
> *a wake-up call to remember*
> *that twenty-four soccer games*
> *and twenty-four soccer practices*
> *in eight weeks is a blessing, not a curse,*
> *even if they are on Sunday.*
>
> *So, Lord, feel free to rock my world,*
> *rotate my axis, shake these bones,*
> *rattle the cage, and liberate my joy.*
> *Behold, the sun does rise on the Monday,*
> *after all three soccer games in the park.*

As Alex predicted, the schools were great for the children, and the soccer fields were less than two miles away. He was home every night for supper, as promised, but had to read and research for hours afterwards. Life was simple and sweet except for my homesickness. Working in a rural area had its challenges; there was no child psychiatrist for collaboration. Since I had to call my attending physician at the Children's Hospital in Virginia for the most complicated cases, my supervision was long distance.

Gradually, the diagnostician in me noticed how much things bothered me in the dark of winter. Summer came, and I seemed better able to cope with life's ups and downs. I was strong and energetic. In October, I was dragging. By November, getting to the dry cleaners or the grocery store seemed like climbing a steep mountain. Fortunately, my new supervisor and I talked weekly—by telephone since he lived two hours away.

One Tuesday morning, during our conversation, he diagnosed me with winter blues.

"Many people at this latitude have it, Julia. I think you should try a light box. Call The SunBox® and get a recommendation. They offer support, research, and many books about the subject. Read *Winter Blues* by Norman Rosenthal, a researcher in mood disorders, at the National Institute of Health, who suffered from seasonal affective disorder (SAD). After realizing he was unable to meet his grant application deadlines in the winter, he investigated and became a pioneer in the field of seasonal depression."

The light box was delivered two days later. Sitting under it for thirty minutes in the morning and thirty minutes in the early evening changed my life. I regained my energy and positive outlook. My time management and organization skills resurfaced. I noticed a difference in my gross and fine motor skills on the tennis court—I could hit the ball and run!

The whole family started the day under a large sun light flooding the breakfast area. Even the children seemed to bicker less after the sun box arrived, and there were no side effects.

Despite the adjustment problems, losses, and trauma stories—or perhaps, because of them—I began spending Fridays at an Episcopal convent, a few months after we opened the RTF. I left home as soon as the children were in school, and returned in time to pick them up. In between, I meditated and communed with the nuns and priest. We shared morning and noonday prayer and ate in silence.

The convent was set on a hill, surrounded by lovingly tended gardens. The priest at the convent offered spiritual direction, and we met weekly. He heard my stories, and together we prayed.

Sharing my anger, I said, "It's as if he isn't listening and doesn't care. How could God have created this mess?"

My new habit became praising God while ranting about sexual perversions.

Meanwhile, the routine at work was growing more onerous. Giving up my private practice, which I loved, to make room for all the demands of the agency, created a gap. I missed adult patients.

"Mom, why did you quit the job you like and work more in the job you don't like?" Jack said.

Marveling at his insight, and not having a good answer, I laughed.

POOL

*I got through it by turning to God,
and forgave my tormentor to help myself heal.
I'm tired of holding this in.
I don't know what to do with it anymore,
so I've decided to give some away.*

—Tyler Perry

"Hey, Dr. Burns, come play pool with us!"

Hector and Joe were rivals. Everybody knew to stay clear when those two were engaged in a pool match. Residents weren't allowed to bet, but it was well-known that they traded each other in chores and clean-up duties.

I was late for a meeting and had two psychiatric evaluations to proof, as well as a new admission coming in that afternoon. Lab values were expected soon, and a female patient needed monitoring. We had stopped her Depakote® because her liver functions had deteriorated, and we were hoping for improvement. There was never a good time to play pool, but I turned around and headed back to the recreation area.

"I'll take the loser," I said.

"Loser? Dr. Burns, you always take loser," Hector said. "That's stupid. Why don't you just do what everyone else does and take winner? I'm going to win, and I want to play you. If you keep doing that, then one time I'm going to have to lose on purpose, and that will destroy my winning streak. Come on, Dr. Burns, don't be an idiot."

Stupid and *idio*t were not supposed to be said in the unit, but for the sake of peace and camaraderie, I chose to disregard it.

"I'll choose whomever I want, and I choose loser."

A lousy pool player, I knew that to take on Hector would have been the shortest game in history. He could rack the table on one turn. Plus, he was fun to tease.

"I'll play you tomorrow, win or lose," I said.

This satisfied him, and the games began. A few minutes later, I was heading down the hall to my office, the workload on my mind.

"Dr. Burns, I need to talk to you about Sheila," said Bill, one of our social workers. "She's not eating again, and the staff believes that the smell in her room is from her hiding her feces. Her treatment team meeting is not for another three weeks. Can we brainstorm some new behavioral management techniques for eating and hoarding today? That way, I can have measurements of success when the team gathers."

Sheila had become so much more socialized since her admission to the RTF. She was showering and dressing on her own. Able to go to the on-grounds school, she completed small academic assignments. Her time-outs in the quiet room had decreased from two, to three a day, to once or twice a week. Only her hoarding, hiding feces, and purging after meals remained problems. The treatment team had been attempting to phase out these maladaptive behaviors for three months, with only intermittent success.

"Sure, Bill, come on in. I've got some psychiatric evals to review, but they can wait."

Bill was a favorite of mine and of many patients. He was compassionate and organized. Never afraid to set limits if necessary, he knew when to pull back and let patients find their way.

Sheila needed a firmer and more precise behavioral plan. Thirty minutes later, Bill and I had new treatment goals with specific consequences for destructive behaviors.

"Let's see how she does with these new incentives. Also, don't forget to ask Sheila what rewards she would like for safe behavior. The girls are getting manicures next week. Or perhaps the recreation therapist could work with her one-on-one."

Often, no matter how we tried to coax and reinforce normal behaviors, the patients would remain attached to their dysfunctional habits. They felt safest staying the same. Change was scary and came slowly, even when the maladaptive behaviors caused significant harm. Bill understood the need for gradual transitions.

Finally, able to read and edit the psychiatric evaluations that had been completed last week, I reviewed Johnny and Jim's story. As brothers, they fiercely protected each other against the abuse of their mother and her boyfriends.

JOHNNY

Suffocating in a web of deceit and violence,
these brothers saw no way out.
Writing late into the night,
I could feel their song weaving a black strand,
blacker net, blackest dark around my slumber.
Let my own children sleep unencumbered, I
prayed, as I wove this song by moonlight's note.
Shadowy webs in the darkness encircle our castle,
hold forever fast this singer, her players,
their stories, and all who listen.
—Julia W. Burns, MD

BOTH JOHNNY AND HIS BROTHER JIM were admitted to the treatment facility the same week. The report read something like this:

Johnny is an eight-year-old African-American male who came to our residential treatment center after being charged with shoplifting at a convenience store. During the initial psychiatric evaluation, he revealed that he only stole if there was no food in the house. When his mother was high on crack, Johnny made sure no one went hungry. His mental status exam revealed that Johnny was a fighter. His IQ was below average, and despite his intellectual challenges, he knew when his mother sold their food stamps that the money was going to drugs, not supper. It was then that he would forage into convenience stores and grocery stores—wherever the boys could walk—and lift packs of crackers, cookies, soda—any small item they could hide inside their coats to stave off starvation. He was hyperactive, hyper-aroused, inattentive, distracted, and aggressive verbally and physically. As a result, Johnny had difficulty learning and behaving in school.

"Dr. Burns, the labs just came," Cynthia said. "You better review them. It looks like Patsy's liver function tests are not normalizing."

"Thanks, Cynthia. Come in. I'm reviewing Jim and Johnny's psychiatric evaluation. What a life they've had." I looked up from my work.

Cynthia was our charge nurse; she typically knew what I was looking for, and was there to assist me and could manage the drama on the unit, including talking down an angry adolescent.

"Yes," Cynthia said. "Johnny is having a tough time following the rules. He gets violent when we try to get him to school. The staff is discouraged. We are waiting for your evaluation so we can call an emergency treatment team meeting. One of our childcare workers got kicked hard this morning."

"I'm finishing it now, and they can read it tonight so we can meet tomorrow. Make sure Dr. Smith knows to come. We will need everyone's input to minimize injuries."

"Oh, Dr. Burns, I know I haven't done right by these boys," the mother said, during the intake. "I've had my problems. My father left us when I was little, and my mother, she was so fragile, she couldn't take care of us. Mom's boyfriends and drug dealers abused us, all of us, the boys and the girls. She took in one man after another, hoping the next one would be different. They were all the same, hurting her during the day and us at night. Foster care was not much better. There were five of us and they split us up. By then, I was so angry that I hit the other foster kids. That got me kicked out and around until I didn't know where to go after school."

This mother had never known a safe home. She had lived in fourteen foster homes, frequently removed because of her inappropriate behavior. It seemed that sexual abuse occurred in the birth home and in her foster placements. Heroin was all she lived for, and hooking for drugs was the path. She gave her boys the same home life her mother had given her. They had been exposed to multiple boyfriends, pimps, and drug dealers as well. Pushed aside and abused, the boys vacillated between numb and enraged, and in her drug-induced stupor, the mother remained indifferent.

Jim was the cute, smart brother. Johnny was the scapegoat. His mother was quick to target him with her wrath. If the electricity was turned off, he was beaten for forgetting to "mail the check." If there was no food and the younger children were crying, it was his fault for neglecting them. If the crack or heroin delivery was late, Johnny was placed in the corner to stand until the dealer showed. If the apartment was dirty, it was his turn to clean. She beat him when he wet his bed and forgot to change the sheets. Johnny's life was hard, and he took the blame to protect his three younger siblings.

By the time Johnny and I met, anger smoldered beneath his dark brown eyes, reflecting the inequity of his eight years. He was haunted by shame and inadequacy. This combined to create a boy who was mannered and thoughtful when things were going his way. But if asked to transition from playtime on the rug to math, violence erupted. His teachers were confused by the severity of his aggression, the suddenness of his mood changes. Johnny would hit the student next to him, throw a book, or stab himself with his pencil. He re-created any number of abusive experiences.

"Dr. Burns, we can't predict his outbursts," said Tom, a childcare worker. "He blows up seconds after he's been laughing and having fun. There doesn't seem to be any precipitant to the rage he shows."

"Let's give Dr. Smith a chance to put together a behavioral program for Johnny. How many mornings is he aggressive before school?"

"Every morning, Dr. Burns. I'm telling you, it's bad. We have a problem. Did you hear that Pat had to file an incident report and leave work yesterday?"

"Yes. Let's try to convince Johnny that if he can go to school one to two days a week without kicking or throwing an object, that he gets to play pool outside of rec time. Dr. Smith, why don't you meet with him and see what other incentives he'd enjoy. Also, let's assign only seasoned, non-confrontational childcare workers. Try to ascertain if he does better with two workers or one, male or female. After an attack, go back at least one hour and examine every ten-minute interval for any changes. I think this is a good start. When do you want to reconvene?"

"Tomorrow," one worker volunteered quickly.

"How about two days?" Candy, Johnny's therapist suggested.

My team had worked with me for a while. We all understood that fear was Johnny's guide. Fear led him to paranoia, violence, and physical destruction. Often, he would be so overwhelmed by adrenaline and cortisol that he would not remember his episodes.

"Johnny, do you know what got you so upset that you kicked Pat?"

"I didn't kick him, Dr. Burns," he usually replied.

We continued to meet frequently, and struggled with Johnny's treatment. Great difficulty lies in teaching a child about anger management if he cannot remember the events leading up to his aggression; impossible to ask him to name his triggers if he blacks out as soon as his rage takes over.

Gradually, we discovered that additional chores and responsibility for younger patients calmed him. We put him in charge of organizing the recreation room for activities. With supervision, he was allowed to lead art projects with younger patients. We shared this treatment approach with his teacher, and soon he began to enjoy school more. Being in charge gave him a sense of security that kept everyone safe.

JIM

*A sibling may be the keeper of one's identity,
the only person with the keys
to one's unfettered, more fundamental self.*
—Marian Sandmaier

JIM'S IQ ON THE OTHER HAND WAS ABOVE AVERAGE, and he learned easily. He solved complicated math problems swiftly, and was reading two levels above his grade. Born to the same mother by different fathers, one could not help but marvel at their intellectual and behavioral differences. Jim was exposed to crack and cocaine in the womb, causing him to be agitated and irritable, as well as inattentive. Wiry and hyperactive, Jim's intelligence allowed him to thrive in the academic setting once Ritalin was prescribed. His inattention and other symptoms responded well to the combination of medication and a therapeutic environment. His ability to learn, juxtaposed with his keen desire to please, allowed him to accelerate academically.

After three months of doing well, he was transferred to a public school, where he continued to follow teachers' instructions and interact appropriately with his peers. He started to trust others not to hurt him, and so gradually responded calmly to authority.

Then suddenly, Jim began to show disruptive behavior. He reverted to pre-medication actions as if he were not taking his Ritalin. He was not physically aggressive, but he became restless and inattentive and acted-out impulsively, touching peers. In-school suspension was applied, but did not decrease the negative behaviors. A special conference was scheduled and included Jim's teacher, nurse, psychologist, and parent.

On the way to that conference, a childcare worker, Robert, said, "Dr. Burns, Dr. Burns, why did you discontinue Jim's Ritalin? He is so much worse without it."

I looked at Robert. He was agitated, his pupils dilated. He had missed the last two monthly medication management appointments, and had failed to provide behavioral information, despite this being mandatory.

He was adamant: "Dr. Burns, you have to restart the Ritalin. I think he would benefit from three times a day, not two."

I reminded him that I had discontinued the Ritalin because it had become ineffective. "Jim's behavior deteriorated weeks before I stopped the medication. It's been harder to evaluate his behavior since you've missed the last two medication reviews, Robert."

He argued with me about this, and I excused myself and headed toward the administrative building, wondering why he had run after me so intently, demanding that the medicine be prescribed. It was rare for childcare workers to argue with doctors, and it struck me that Jim's behavior had declined in conjunction with the childcare worker's.

As I climbed the stairs to the meeting, it occurred to me that perhaps the Ritalin was being diverted—maybe someone was selling it or using it. Someone other than Jim. Robert's agitation, dilated pupils, and perseveration were troubling. Medication reviews were a primary responsibility of the senior childcare workers, and he was missing them.

We spent over an hour in that conference reviewing Jim's case, and decided to restart the Ritalin. I suggested that the nursing department oversee medication administration for one month, under the pretext that Jim needed close supervision in case he was spitting it out. But I told the charge nurse my suspicion that perhaps the medicine was being diverted. She concurred with my assessment of Robert's recent declining work performance, and as we parted she promised to keep a closer eye on him. Immediately, Jim's restless, hyperactive, impulsive behavior ceased. He was able to attend to lessons and complete school assignments and homework easily.

At our next session, Jim proudly said, "Hey, Dr. Burns, I made an 'A' in math today, and I earned the highest behavioral level. I'm doing good again."

"Fantastic, Jim. I'm so proud of you," I said. "What do you think made the difference?"

"I like taking my medicine. It helps me be smarter," he replied, quietly.

"Well, great. We will continue you on the same dose."

He began having fun with his friends again. Talking back to the teacher ceased.

Controlled substances and other medications were bubble packed, making tracking easier. We closely monitored the amount of Ritalin and other stimulants going in and out of the cottage. Under closer inspection, it was discovered that Robert was taking the stimulants. Never sure if he was using or selling, he could no longer handle medication, but was allowed to continue as a childcare worker.

BETRAYAL

In reality, women have always greeted the burden of motherhood ambivalently, even in the best of circumstances, and many women bear children involuntarily. But the opprobrium which attaches to any woman who willingly gives up her child is so great that some mothers will keep and mistreat their children rather than admit that they cannot care for them.
—Judith Lewis Herman

MEANWHILE, AFTER A PERIOD OF RESPONDING to the therapeutic milieu and medication, Johnny began deteriorating. He experienced paranoid delusions that people were talking and laughing at him. Voices haunted him, calling his name and mocking him. He developed a facial tic and head jerk. The genetic history of his father was unknown, but the signs of bipolar disorder—including mood swings, aggression, pressured speech, and paranoid ideation—indicated that Johnny was having a manic episode, with psychotic features complicated by motor tics.

His mother visited the boys every two to three months. She had younger children at home, and the facility was off the bus line, making visitation difficult. Having always been unreliable or abusive, now her presence was virtually nonexistent. And yet

Johnny obsessed about his mother and worried fiercely when she failed to show for scheduled visitations.

"Dr. Burns, my mom is coming this weekend. Did you know that, Dr. Burns? Did you want to come and see her when she visits? Did you know she is bringing me a present? I hope she's bringing something good."

Recently, she had begun participating in a methadone program. Her drug tests had been clean for three months.

As Johnny's symptoms worsened, a trial of oxcarbazepine, a seizure medication known to be effective with mood disorders, was started. It stabilized the violence and diminished the fears. Almost miraculously, Johnny started participating in school activities again, and displayed independence in his daily activities. The childcare workers and clinical staff were relieved as they charted his progress. He was able to complete third grade and move on to fourth grade. A behavioral plan aimed at listening and supporting—but not encouraging—his paranoia was put in place. Johnny maintained his treatment goals under this guidance.

Despite the risks, discharge home was the long-range goal. Plans to incorporate Johnny's mother into treatment began. First, she would visit the cottage at evening meals. Next, Jim and Johnny would have day visits at home, and finally, weekend visits would begin.

Their mother was scheduled to come to the evening meal next Saturday. It was all that Johnny and Jim could speak about.

"Dr. Burns, my mom's coming," Johnny said. "Did you hear? Dr. Burns, do you want to come Saturday? We're having spaghetti, my mom's favorite. Are you coming, Dr. Burns?"

"I'll look forward to hearing about it on Monday," I said, "and I'll see your mother in the treatment team meeting next week."

I saw him sooner. When his mom failed to come for supper, he went on a rampage, breaking pool cues and threatening workers. With the strength of his adrenaline surge,

Johnny demolished the lounge, cursing as he lifted and flipped the sofa. The details of his aggressive acts were described to me as I listened that Saturday evening.

"Dr. Burns, he ran outside, not to hide in the cemetery as he often does, but to break windows. He brought the pool cue outside and started beating the brick. He wasn't able to break any windows, but he did smash several frames."

"Is anyone hurt? Don't go near him. Keep him in eyesight, but stay at least twelve feet away. Follow him if he tries to head down the highway. He is in no shape to be wandering alone. But do not corner him."

"Of course, Dr. Burns. We'll stay with him. We won't antagonize him, but we won't allow him to run off."

"Call me back in fifteen minutes, and if he hasn't come inside, I'll come in."

They had no recourse but to force him back into the building and subdue him in the time-out room.

Later, I said, "Johnny, how are you? What happened?"

He could not speak of his mother or her absence, instead blaming another patient who was laughing at him during a pool game.

"You know, Dr. Burns, I'm terrible at pool, but I hate being laughed at."

We did not speak of the missed visit. He was so hurt by her continued betrayal that he probably knew why he was angry, but could not speak of it. Johnny showed a pattern common with children in residential care—escalating aggression with family disappointments.

When a parent repeatedly betrayed a resident, staff felt a keen sense of impotence. One of the ways they tried to overcome their negative feelings was to fantasize about rescuing the children. Jim was endearing, so beloved that some staff approached me about fostering him with the goal of adoption.

"Dr. Burns, I told my husband about Jim, and we think we could make a good home for him. The girls are four and six now, and could use an older brother."

Jim had been in our care for three years. Terminating parental rights had failed in the past. The mother became active and resistant to termination when adoptive parents were identified.

"Karen, don't you remember that Jim was sexually molested in his mother's home? That he came to White Pines after failing three foster placements because of inappropriate sexual behaviors?"

Also, Jim and another boy allegedly had oral sex in the cottage, continuing this behavior despite multiple interventions.

We discussed a recent sexual abuse incident in the home of a White Pines social worker.

"Don't you remember that Charles fostered a male resident and the trauma history was not reviewed?" I said. "The boy sexually abused his three children. Consider your best work done here at White Pines and not in your home until your girls are much older."

She agreed, reluctantly. Jim and Johnny continued to be favorites among the staff and were never able to return home. After a protracted stay at White Pines, Jim was discharged to foster care, and Johnny to a lower level of residential care. Although his mother never showed the capacity to care for them consistently, the boys still loved her. She loved them, too, even though her treatment of them interfered with their safety and well-being.

Unfortunately, generations of neglect and abuse create parental patterns that repeat the traumatic cycle. Without interventions, they, just like their children, impulsively act on their violent rages, repeatedly inflicting the harsh punishments they themselves are so desperate to escape.

SOMEBODY

If only we could escape from this house of incest,
where we only have ourselves in the other,
if only I could save you all from yourselves.
—Anais Nin

I SING A SONG OF THE INCESTUAL RELATIONSHIP between a daughter, Sandra, and her stepfather. She lies in panic, waiting for him to come home—every night. When he violates her, she dissociates, riding the crest of an atmospheric wave far away where she sings on a star, another song, a song of hope, and a different life. Dreaming of her future, she escapes the weight of this grown man lying on her, squeezing her breath and snuffing out the life she should be living.

Somebody is hiding.
She lies there, her body wedged tight,
lidless eyes press into ironed white sheets.
Tiny pink lines, stripes sever wide white intervals.
Someone else is home, too.
Sandra hides behind this curtain, invisible,
as spirits hover and view her beating terror.

A father enters,
though the dresser barricades the opening:
six drawers arise, erect sentries guarding the secret.

  The girl conceals her body.

  She is hiding. She is home.

Light filters through the crack, pink tattered
 wallflower exposed as the door groans,
and he plunges into a hole far too fine.

As he finds the almost invisible under the pink and
 white ironed linens that veil her, she flees.

Fly with her, fly as he unfastens her body.

Depart as the angels fiercely surround the
 separation, enduring this hidden life.

  Spin out, out thin and beyond,
  sleep blown backward.

  Sway away, east lies west.

Disconnect from his entry, as a filter of golden
thread spins you away and you fly with Sandra.

 The ladder runs from moonbeam
to garbage dump, return ticket paid in full,
 but whirl now into the wider air.

Sky-fly past the television where her brother lies,
 watching as another detective
  drops his bullet again,
where Mother lies sleeping, curled in half,
 blank bitterness her only bedfellow.

Divide into vapors that flatten as they splay away.

Climb higher than the blades, the lying backpack
 and dresser leaning against the door,
the TV's hum, and green leaves' vibrations.

 Hang upside down in their rhythm,
swing on the handle of the Big Dipper.

Sing broken lyrics with fish on a star,
and let the song sway, the musical roar separate
and sustain the hidden whole.

In the distance, each silent scream reverberates
as shattered fragments scatter.

Somebody is hiding. Someone else is home.

Now lying in cooling drool, laden oozing.

Ironed sheets, pink, thin lines
sever clean white spaces.

She lives in there.
Bite her and she bleeds.

Sandra was a blonde eight-year-old waif of a girl who entered my office one December after being taken from her parents because of neglect. She was humping children on the playground and in bathrooms, and a teacher reported her behavior to social services, where someone suspected sexual abuse. Although she had seen several therapists and psychiatrists, she refused to talk. She would only play quietly on the floor or sit politely in a chair, refusing to speak. No matter how many providers asked her if she were safe, if anyone was hurting her, the little girl just sat and smiled.

She was well-behaved that day in my office, too. Playing with the toys on the rug, seeking approval for every movement. I gave this readily, knowing the only way to gain entry to her secret world was to observe her without judgment or speech. She moved from playing on the rug to jumping in my lap, thrusting her hips toward mine. I calmly moved her back to the play area without a word. Quizzically, she gazed at me and sashayed toward the door as if to leave. Once more, I refrained from correction, determined to follow her and transcribe her reactions.

Instead of walking away, she started sucking the door knob. She gyrated and sucked the knob of my office door for many long minutes, putting the whole doorknob in her mouth. After that, she began licking the door hinges, her provocative sexual dance continuing—her story coming to light as I watched. This time, the one who said nothing was me. There were no words for what I was witnessing as she moved to the chalkboard, and while gyrating up and down, licked it clean.

This took over an hour, as it was a large black chalkboard, and she licked every inch. Every few minutes, she would pause and glance my way, wondering if I was watching, if I cared, if I was going to ask her to stop, or perhaps tell her to thrust her hips a bit more to the left.

Although neither of us said a word, it was one of the most difficult psychiatric interviews I have ever done. After escorting her back to the nursing office, where her foster parents were waiting, I came out of the office, looking ashen.

Joan, my nurse said, "Dr. Burns, are you OK?"

I nodded. "Yes. Please wash the doorknob and chalkboard. I am going for a walk."

I could not talk or tell the story I had just seen. Instead, I went outside for fresh air, nauseous, circling the block slowly while Joan cleaned the office.

I wrote Sandra's report, describing her sexualized behavior: "Sandra presents as a clean, small, white female who appears younger than her stated age of eight. Although she was mute during the interview, her behavior was aggressively sexual. The patient tried to initiate a lap dance, but was easily redirected to the toys on the floor. Completely non-verbal during her pornographic performance, her intent was clear."

Describing her actions allowed social services to place her at White Pines.

Why do we allow children to be sexualized and abused simply because we don't want to think about trauma, choosing to remain uneducated and unmoved despite the statistics? Silent observers are as active as perpetrators when they step aside, letting priests, principals, teachers, janitors, neighbors, coaches, scout leaders, relatives, and parents molest children or create child pornography.

In my lectures about sexual abuse, I often remind staff that we have created a culture that elevates sex in all forms of media—music, movies, advertising, and magazines—with little regard for the consequences to children.

"Last week," I said, "I was called to consult with a school, regarding the suspension of an eleven-year-old boy. When angered by the teacher, he responded, 'Get down on your knees and suck me.' The teacher was astonished. I'm not, and you shouldn't be either. This vocabulary is common fare in children's mainstream music and movies. Film directors, actors, and musicians who include graphic sexual material in their creations are perpetrators. When we fail to safeguard children, we are enablers."

Encouraging childcare workers and teachers to be watchful for abusers within their agency, families, and neighborhoods, my work to educate parents, patients, and childcare workers was relentless. But so was my growing sense that childhood trauma could be eliminated. Identifying with my patients so much that their symptoms became mine, I suffered my own trauma in listening to theirs. But it was my angry accusations against God that wounded me most.

Social services often investigated and came away with too little evidence, or the child recanted in fear. Often, children were placed in foster or adoptive homes, only to be abused in that environment, too. Child protective workers and law enforcement officers failed to find evidence in cases of child abuse, repeatedly stepping aside so that perpetrators gained easy access. This act of omission opened a path for perpetrators who cannot self-regulate, and required others to be the watch dog for them. Children such as Sandra saw that they would not be protected, so they learned not to trust. No wonder children remained silent. No wonder there are so few dialogues with victims about their abuse. Thank goodness for that doorknob and chalkboard. Thank goodness for a little girl who spoke loudly without words, and for a doctor who watched and documented what she saw.

The next day, I saw the psychologist who also evaluated Sandra. I asked her what she thought.

She replied, "Not much. She wouldn't speak."

I said, "Didn't she try to hump you?"

"Oh, that. Yes, she did, but I told her to get down, that she was naughty."

"Did she stop?"

"Yes, but that was it."

Of course, it was. And I stood there in disbelief, both hers and mine. Did it really happen? Did I sit in a chair and watch a young girl suck a door knob and gyrate and then lick an enormous chalkboard? If no one else sees these things, hears these stories, are they true? Because what is truth but a collective experience, an emergence of theory in accordance with fact or reality?

Why, I asked for the millionth time was my reality so different from others? And a wall, dense as concrete, slammed down between us so that I stood in impenetrable isolation. It was the isolation as much as the stories that created the burnout. The depravity of the patient's stories was so intense that speaking these atrocities out loud was impossible.

I was a prisoner in my own life.

HENRY

*Here's another old saying
that deserves a second look:
'Eye for eye, tooth for tooth.'
Is that going to get us anywhere?
Here's what I propose:
'Don't hit back at all.'*
—Matthew 5:38-28

HENRY WAS FIFTEEN AND A HALF when he was seen on a Person in Need of Supervision (PINS) petition because of his academic failure, truancy, and oppositional behavior. He had been out of treatment since his discharge from White Pines at age eight. I often thought we were too late for some of our patients. This time, it proved true.

At age sixteen, teenagers can become emancipated minors, legally independent, making treatment plans less relevant. Patients can then make choices about whether to go to school or take medication, and where they want to live. Henry was certain about dropping out of school: "I failed first grade, and I've hated it ever since."

His mother admitted to a long history of neglect and abuse: "I was able to care for his sister, but I could not stand Henry. My mother came to assist with his care when he was born to prevent placement with the county."

He had low weight gain and repeated hospitalizations due to bronchial infections. Diagnosed with Failure to Thrive, Child Protective Services noted that he was "malnourished as an infant, investigation closed." His mother broke his clavicle when he was five, and the county placed him in foster care for about eight months. She took a parent-training class so he could return to the home, but how do you teach an abusive, neglectful mother to love, especially when she had never known love herself?

> *They both heard the crack his clavicle made*
> *when it shattered, broken by his flight,*
> *propelled into the air by rage, wrath spilling out,*
> *ripping, and lifting him into the wall.*
>
> *He splintered.*
>
> *How long ago were her bones cracked*
> *by her mother?*
>
> *Generational neuronal configurations*
> *dug deep in grooves of rage so that nobody forgets*
> *when it's time to throw the next baby*
> *against the wall.*
>
> *Both living with busted bones, shattered dreams,*
> *splintered pieces left for the doctor to mend.*
>
> *In looking for love, they repeat a pattern deep,*
> *dug in, and stuck in the only groove they know.*
>
> *After she threw him, they traveled to the*
> *orthopedist, but when she dragged him*
> *across the waiting room,*
> *he screamed, trembled, and cowered.*
>
> *And so child protective services was called*
> *—"clavicle broken, mother grabbed him by*
> *the arm and roughly pulled him, odorous and*
> *unkempt."*
>
> *Who picked him up and brought him to me?*

*I wish I remembered, because that's how I came
to know a small boy with a broken clavicle,
who trembled when he walked
because he worried about walls falling in
and breaking him to pieces all the time.*

"I began to like him a little bit when he was three, but it wasn't until he was eight years old—after his first stay at White Pines and his father taking custody—that we bonded." His mother repeated her story, as I asked questions.

Eight years is a long time to be unloved by your mother.

Henry was discharged from White Pines to his biological father's home, and he stayed there despite constant physical abuse. Henry was a bed-wetter and was beaten on his back and legs with belts, sticks, hands, "whatever his father had." He was forced to sit in his bedroom, facing the wall, for up to six hours at a time. When I asked Henry why he never told the judge or his mother about the punishments, he gave a frequently heard answer: "I didn't know there was anything wrong with it."

Finally, his sister had visitation, and when she returned from the father's house with welts, his mother tried to regain custody of Henry.

His diagnostic evaluation read as follows:

> *There is inattention, hyperactivity, impulsivity, and poor organization. Henry loses things, is forgetful, and distracted. He is noncompliant with medication for attention-deficit/hyperactivity disorder, and his mother does not enforce compliance. Her depression keeps her from being an effective parent. Henry began to experiment with marijuana after failing eighth grade the second time. He felt nothing could be gained from attending school, so he didn't go. He left his mother's house and is living in a one-*

bedroom apartment with an adult male friend of the family.

Henry plans to drop out of school in three months and is interested in construction. He is courageous, humorous, and honest. He has never tried to kill himself, but a year ago he stated, "I wished I'd never been born, and I'll never say again 'what a big deal that was.'"

Research shows that children who are not nurtured, loved, held, stimulated, and fed show increased incidences of learning and behavioral disorders. The school should have developed an Individualized Education Plan (IEP) for Henry in first grade given his math difficulties and academic failure overall. Wellbutrin XL may be a good choice for Henry to treat his ADHD and anger. However, compliance in a teenager who is living away from home is questionable.

If the home he is living in is safe and drug free, that would be good. However, many abused children lie about the safety of their living situation because they are fearful. Henry's lack of experience with normal, nurturing homes makes it possible that he has put himself into a dangerous situation. The department of social services should assess this home.

Alternatively, there is no evidence to support improvement in the family's functioning should Henry return home. His strengths are his interests in mechanics and construction. He is not currently using drugs. He is handsome and funny. He has no criminal record. He wants to support himself.

Impressed with Henry's courage, I sat and listened to and loved the child no one else had loved, hearing tales of abuse, of staring at the wall for hours, of beatings and bruises, with his not knowing those were wrong. He had no idea that life could be different, and he never wondered if the little boy sitting beside him at school went home to hugs, milk, and cookies.

After Henry left, I completed my report. Reminding God of these broken lives, my hurting patients, my sorrow-filled parents, I questioned him again: Are you watching this Lord? What are you doing to make it better?

I heard this answer: *Ask parents in labor and delivery, If you aren't going to feed this child, hold this child, and protect him, can we find him another family?*

And so many of my families, knowing their broken lives, would answer, "Yes, take this child. Have someone else raise him, because I can't. But I'd like to visit. Can I?"

Why can't we answer, "Yes, that's possible? Open adoption is a possibility for this child."

Three years later, I was interviewed by a state attorney seeking mitigation for Henry, against the death penalty. Henry and his cousin were incarcerated for killing a policeman. They were robbing a convenience store when a policeman surprised them and the cousin shot him. Henry told them, "I didn't even have a gun."

While reviewing his history with the attorney, and knowing that his mother could not feed him or love him, that his father beat him for bed-wetting, I said, "Henry failed first grade once and eighth grade twice, and never learned to read."

"Yes," said the lawyer, "abuse is a mitigating factor. But did he also have a head injury? Is he mentally retarded?"

Finally, someone was paying attention. It must have felt good to Henry that his lawyer was trying to help, even though his primary goal was to defeat the death penalty, not assist Henry.

I didn't cry when I was notified of his sentence—life in prison. By then, it was too late for me, too. I'd been working at White Pines for four years, and the numbness of my secondary trauma had taken roots. Shutting down my emotions in an effort to survive every day had become a tool in my repertoire, too.

DO YOU FEEL SAFE?

> *He heals the heartbroken*
> *and bandages their wounds.*
>
> —Psalm 147:3

PATIENTS TEASED ME ON MORNING ROUNDS. "Dr. Burns, do you feel safe?" they said, parroting my question to them every morning and after each episode of violence.

"What happened, Jesse? Did you feel safe when you got angry and threw the scissors?" I would ask.

But by the end of 1998, my patients, my staff, knew something was wrong. They watched as I entered their rooms early in the morning, checking mental status and behavioral levels. I was absent, much the same way they were after a flashback. We struggled to connect. Although they continued to look to me for stability and safety, we witnessed a shift in my ability to provide it. No one spoke it out loud, but everyone knew I was struggling. The abuse stories and my patients' pain, the administration's position on extra staffing for the cottages at night, the twenty-four-hour on-call schedule, and our inability to stabilize the childcare staff and create a therapeutic milieu, all began to take its toll.

"Dr. Burns, we're ordering pizza for the staff meeting. Are you in?" Mel the cook said, trying to feed me back to health. "Or I'll make macaroni and cheese instead, if you want."

"Dr. Burns, I wrote this poem about you," Patty said. "Can I read it? It's better than yours."

"Dr. Burns, look at this red tulip I painted for you," Carrie said. "Do you like it?"

The caretaking extended across both sides of the table. I increased staff trainings and worked hard with social workers to create dynamic treatment plans for difficult patients. Efforts to establish a therapeutic milieu that would create healing were vital, and yet many days it felt as if we were all failing. I spent much time planning and executing lectures on verbal and physical aggression, dissociation, and flashbacks common with PTSD. We made connections to patients' abuse and how that informed their aggression. Initially, staff seemed grateful and tried hard to comply with protocols to reduce aggression and increase safety. More recently, I despaired that the trainings were falling on deaf ears, as childcare workers lived below the poverty level, and staff turnover, which contributed to inexperience, was constant.

Why had the childcare workers allowed the adolescents to watch *Freddy Krueger* when it was on the no-watch list?

"Dr. Burns, don't worry. It was the edited version," said Carter, our senior childcare worker.

"What difference could that possibly make?" I said. "*No watch* means no, never, they cannot watch it. They are weaned on *Freddy Krueger* and *Friday the 13th*. Their perpetrators use these movies to intimidate and control them through fear, and then seduce them. They beg to watch horror flicks in an effort to prove that they are brave enough to survive. Don't you remember the training we had on this last month? You'll have to take my word for it that horror movies re-create trauma."

I was angry, but I soon forgot the disagreement in light of the party planned for Barbie's birthday. The surprise was not actually for Barbie, but for our manager of operations, John. Over the years, John had become increasingly close to Barbie. He would find that little doll on his work cart and in the bathroom, sitting on a pipe that required replacing. She could be seen in the lunchroom, claiming the chair beside his. Barbie sometimes came to treatment teams or staff meetings to tell us how wonderful John was and what a great job he was doing. Barbie's affection for John had grown over the years, till she was the mascot, practical joker, and chief beauty queen for the RTF.

Rob, one of the social workers, had started the prank three years ago and never let up. Barbie could be found anywhere at any time, and today was her special day. Mel cooked hot dogs, salad, broccoli, and a pink cake for the party, and Rob hid Barbie in the kitchen. We asked John to come to the kitchen to check a faulty burner on the stove.

While John was busy examining the stove, I said, "Hey John, have you seen Barbie? It's her special day, and we have a surprise."

"What's so special about today, Dr. Burns? I've got a leaking toilet in room twelve because one of the residents tried to flush another stuffed animal. There's a flood in there, and now Mel interrupts me to check a burner that's working. Nothing special about it, I'm telling you. I don't have time for this foolishness. Somebody has to work around here."

Rob walked over and pulled Barbie out from under the tool box. "Looks like you've got more than work on your mind. Looks like you and Barbie were going swimming. She's wearing her bathing suit."

"It's minus ten degrees, Rob. That's a scary thought, even for you, who likes ice fishing. Get out of here, all of you, grinning like cats, and let me get on with my work."

When he finished his grumbling, out popped Leslie and Mel with the cake, singing "Happy Birthday."

And that's when John really became unglued. "Goldarn it, what's going on around here? Singing, a stove that's working, and the whole treatment team standing around laughing like we don't have eighteen patients who need more attention than I do. You guys are foolish."

So we told him, "Barbie is having a party, and you are her favorite guest."

And that's when he got it. Barbie, the birthday cake, the singing, the fake broken stove, and best of all, the hot dogs. Barbie held us accountable, leading us from dark news and difficult therapy sessions to playfulness. Her ability to pop up, greeting us with her perfect figure and wardrobe, gave us many smiles.

There was so much we were trying to forget.

ALLISON

Go ahead and be angry.
You do well to be angry—but don't use your anger
as fuel for revenge.
And don't stay angry.
Don't go to bed angry.
Don't give the Devil
that kind of foothold in your life.
—Ephesians 4:26-27

CYNTHIA, OUR CHARGE NURSE, stuck her head into my office. "Dr. Burns, your evaluation is here. Remember Allison from the state hospital? Dr. Gaskin called and requested a case review. Are you ready? Should I bring her in?"

After the party that day, we had a team consultation. A young girl who was on the children's unit at the state psychiatric hospital was coming to be interviewed. Her inpatient doctors wanted to discharge her to White Pines, but she was doing so poorly that there was little hope she would be ready for transfer. Our job was to meet her, give her a tour of the facility, and assess our ability to keep her safe at a lower level of care.

Looking up from her chart and sighing, I wondered what trauma could create such behaviors in a small girl. What had she seen in her short life, and what more could I learn after spending two hours interviewing her?

I asked Cynthia, "How can I impact this young girl's life when so many doctors and providers have failed?"

She had no answer, so I got ready to meet Allison, to listen in a new way. I hoped her treatment plan could be altered, and she could decrease the behaviors that got her kicked out of school and foster homes. Her psychiatric record read:

> *Allison is a 9-year-old white female who has a long history of neglect, physical and sexual abuse. Symptoms included verbal aggression, mood lability, sleep disturbance with sleep walking, poor hygiene, fighting with siblings, sexual acting out, and self-injurious behaviors, including picking sores and biting her tongue until it bleeds. Her previous diagnoses include bipolar disorder, Attention-deficit disorder, and oppositional defiant disorder.*

Where is post-traumatic stress disorder, chronic type? I typed her clinical summary:

> *Allison was seen with her biological father—who recently gained custodial care—and his girlfriend. Her father reported severe neglect in the maternal home from zero to two years of age. Allison was frequently found wandering the streets at night. She was removed at the age of two on grounds of neglect. Allison's older sister, four at the time of the children's removal, was the primary caretaker in the family.*
>
> *All the children were exposed to alcohol in utero. And in the home, they were exposed to adult sexual activity. At a young age, they played a game called "dragon or diaper," where the mother's father "peed on them and they had to sip it off." The social service worker noted this seemed to be a reference to oral sex. When Allison was examined, there were*

> *bruises and red marks in the diaper area. Allison had multiple imaginary friends who "play games with her and keep her company late at night when she is afraid."*

It is not unusual for aggressive children to act out only when challenged. A good child psychiatrist is a team member and operates like a tenacious detective, scouring medical records for clues and extracting information about a patient's function—often never seeing the maladaptive behaviors, because even aggressive, hyperaroused children can behave normally under controlled situations.

> *Mental status exam reveals a clean, white female in no apparent distress. Eye contact is good. Speech is of regular rate and rhythm. Thoughts are goal directed. Content centers around missing her mom, but liking it at her dad's house. No auditory or visual hallucinations. No suicidal or homicidal ideation. No thought insertion, broadcasting, or withdrawal. Mood is euthymic. Affect is appropriate. She endorses thoughts of wishing she had never been born. No attempts at suicide. Cognition is intact. She demonstrates abstract thinking. Judgment is fair. Insight is fair. Her response to three wishes is, "Live in New Orleans, live with my grandma, live with my grandpa who is dead, and that's my three wishes."*

And what were my three wishes? I wished Allison had not been abused by her mother's father and her mother's boyfriends. I wished I'd never heard a perpetrator say, "I do it because it's the only time I feel anything. I'm numb except when having sex with children. I know it's wrong. Every time, when it's over, I swear, never again. But then I find myself circling back, hovering, watching, waiting until its bath time. I live only for the next connection."

I can't remember what my third wish was that day, but I'm certain it had to do with God.

Allison was already receiving the maximum level of care at the state psychiatric hospital. As a consultant reviewing her behavioral plan and recommending medication changes, I hoped her aggression would decrease so she could shower without a fight. But what if showers led to sexual molestation for her like they did for so many children? The soap a lubricant for sex, occurring in the bathtub while her older sister watched and waited, knowing she was next. Who was I to speak to her about cleanliness and going to school smelly when she knew what happens when little girls step into the tub? And how could we put that in a treatment plan?

My mind tumbled. What could I do but increase her Depakote, a mood stabilizer, or decrease it and wean her off so we could observe her without medication, and then perhaps start Lithium, another medicine with mood-stabilizing properties?

This little girl cleared the teacher's desk in anger, breaking a favorite coffee mug. She grabbed the crotch of her friend; she didn't know how to play hopscotch, but she knew sex games well. Her individualized treatment plan already included intensive services, individual therapy, cognitive behavioral therapy, and family therapy. What could I possibly add? I reviewed psychoeducational material about bipolar disorder and post-traumatic stress disorder, and we discussed the symptoms of chronic trauma, including dissociation. I attempted to explain the phenomenon of flashbacks—that Allison might not remember her aggression or sexual acting out.

"It's harder for her to take responsibility if she cannot remember," I told her father, counseling patience.

But where were the providers and individualized treatment plans nine and a half years ago when she was born? Born into an addicted, aggressively sexualized family that molested her, forgot to feed her, or lock the front door at night after they passed out, she needed our help then.

Documenting findings and chairing team meetings felt ineffective. Each patient was medicated in hopes of giving them a life without aggression, but I felt trepidation. I wanted them in school where they could learn, but I knew that anger and aggression were their defenses. And so I persisted—writing prescriptions, signing off on treatment plans, and supervising therapists, hoping some good was being created, that healing was occurring.

After six years at White Pines, I was suffering physically and mentally. There was a ringing and fullness in my right ear that irritated me. Rushing through the work day, I rarely had time to eat, and would come home ravenous, grabbing snacks from the pantry to assuage my hunger as I put supper on the table. My knee hurt and buckled when I climbed stairs. Allergies plagued me. Those frigid, sub-zero days when my nose hairs froze and my head pounded from the barometric pressure were exceptionally painful. Bitterness and anger grew as every case revealed maltreatment. I blamed God for Allison's life, and called to him for some meaning in her abuse.

I did not hear an answer. Neither did she.

"Hey, God, listen up. Let's start over. Change creation. Let's counsel Eve about the day the snake came. Let's caution her not to fall for his cunning argument. Let her read a psychiatric evaluation of a six-year-old who was sexually groomed in infancy, tell her about the hundreds of victims that one single perpetrator violates in a lifetime. Please, Lord, tell her before she takes a bite of the apple."

Focusing so much on darkness, I lost sight of the light, lost my faith and joy. Convinced I had to create a trauma-sensitive milieu, then a trauma-sensitive world so abuse could be abolished, I persevered. It was too much to ask, but I couldn't give up, afraid that if I stopped working, things would get worse, that more children would suffer and no one would care. I knew God existed before and outside of time, and that he could fix this, but I didn't believe he would.

God continued loving me during my oppositional outrage. He urged me to see a wider story and asked for a cease fire, but I turned from his goodness. Confused, I felt I couldn't love him and continue listening to my patients, too.

Thus my own secondary post-traumatic stress symptoms were born in this environment of distrust and exhaustion. Some days, I was so distraught over a patient's story or an administrative decision that I was barely present for my own family. This was not the part-time career I had envisioned when I drew a pie chart and chose child psychiatry over OB-GYN.

YOUR SISTER

I stopped reading the paper two years ago,
when the choking began.
The stories lodged tight against my Adam's apple
till I couldn't breathe.
Couldn't sweep the swallow stuck in my throat.
So I stopped reading about them early,
first thing in the morning,
with my green tea and bagel.
Stopped reading so I could pretend
I could breathe at work
when I listened to my children's stories.
But I broke, read about you, little lost boy,
his gun, his fight with a friend on the playground.
Seventeen children filed out to lunch
in a single line, obedient, order well-formed
as he whipped out the barrel, pointed at his
enemy, and then swung and shot her in the neck.
I don't know why I stopped the stopping
and read about you.
Looked at the picture of your mother's
front page weeping in the courtroom.
Read about your father's release from jail to
appear at your side after it happened.

*But even though I read about you,
your mother and father, the flop house and crack,
the policeman who said you didn't stand a chance,
the man who left his gun on your pillow
after he raped your mother,
the little girl who will never go to church again,
her mother who may not either,
the thing I remember most,
can't shake from my brain,
the refrain stuck like the swallow,
"The boy and his brother were placed
with a maternal aunt.
There is a sister, but her location is unknown."*

*So now as I sit in the morning,
not reading the paper again,
I can't help the wondering,*

*How did they lose your sister?
Where is she?
What is her name?*

RESIGNATION

In the Last Days, God says,
I will pour out my Spirit on every kind of people:
Your sons will prophesy, also your daughters;
Your young men will see visions,
your old men dream dreams.

—Acts 2

I WAS JOURNALING AND PRAYING for a different path, seeking a new way to educate people about childhood trauma. The stories, always unique, unfolded as children and teenagers came for medication interviews and psychiatric evaluations. I listened and believed—knowing they were telling the truth. And even though belief was a gift that had rarely been given to them, it wasn't enough. Lacking conviction that any treatment we had to offer would make a permanent difference, hopelessness was my companion. Afraid to go to work and scared to stay home, I, too, was choking—choking on the stories.

I approached our director. "Matt, I'm worried about the supervision of the youngest resident's cottage. Michael, a resident of B Cottage, told me that there is sexual activity at night. He let me know that he and another resident have been 'playing doctor,' and that now it is going further and he is getting scared. I think we should have more than one night worker in a cottage. What do you think?"

Matt agreed that safety was important for the care of each child, but as the conversation turned to the next board meeting and the annual fund, the subject was dropped. If the structure of night supervision in the cottages didn't change and the children were abused in the treatment center, what message did that convey about safety? Wouldn't they view sexual behavior as the norm? My list of reservations over how we were diagnosing and treating trauma was growing.

Most of the time when I was at home, I was free. But not always. More and more, I could hear the echo of my latest forensic testimony about a young boy forced to live outdoors on his screened porch because he destroyed his room. A porta-potty was the only furniture allowed, besides the cot his mother offered. Even on winter nights, he was left to huddle by the kitchen door. He lived this way for over a year, before he went to school and told his teacher. His mother was a teacher also, and this made telling so much more difficult.

Or the girl with cigarette burns all over her body: little circles of red, oozing pus penetrated my vision as I squirted ketchup onto hamburger for the evening's meatloaf. Or the young girl in foster care coming to clinic the next day because she had fondled a younger child. Had the introduction to sex begun in the birth home? Or was the foster home also unsafe?

Emotional numbing, isolation, and cynicism—common symptoms diagnosed in my patients—I now recognized in myself. Each incident reflected in the eyes of a damaged child, an abusive perpetrator, or a silent observer, hurt. Even though I had never heard of it before—because it wasn't recognized yet—I had secondary post-traumatic stress disorder. I couldn't continue to listen.

"I'm burned out, Madeline," I said to the clinical director.

My children, who were three months, three years, and six years when I began my tenure at White Pines, were now six, nine, and twelve years old. I wanted to be home with them, listening to their stories. It was time to resign. I went to work the next day, typed my resignation letter, and handed it to

Madeline, a supportive friend, as well as a crackerjack clinician and administrator.

"Have you told our executive director?" was her only question.

"No, I had to tell you first," I said.

"You have to tell him, Dr. Burns."

When I told Matt, he asked for three to six months to find another doctor. I gave him three.

Immediately, I began to sleep more soundly. I felt more present in my family life, more joyful. The ringing and hearing loss in my right ear began to improve—turned out not listening was good for my hearing. I worried about the difficulties of White Pines finding another child and adolescent psychiatrist, but mostly I was relieved. The "Hallelujah Chorus" rang out several mornings from my office.

"What is that noise?" a visitor asked Cynthia.

"Oh, that? It's Dr. Burns's new routine after morning rounds, playing the 'Hallelujah Chorus.' I wish we were as excited as she is."

The RTF could not continue without a medical director. The patients depended on me as a constant in their lives, one of the few they had ever known. They were certain there would be no one to fill prescriptions, sign treatment-team plans, and play pool in the break room if I left. They had no interest in a new doctor. The staff felt similarly. Mourning began on the day of my resignation, and saturated the next three months.

The childcare workers were also concerned about the transition. They knocked on my door, telling of a patient's defiance, or perhaps someone's successful school day.

"Sandra has gone almost two weeks without eating a light bulb. We are about to decrease her restrictions so she can go off campus. The patients are sad that you are leaving. They've had so many losses. They are talking about it, which is good."

"Yes, we are going to figure out a way to make sure that all treatment, including medications, stay the same for at least six to eight weeks after I leave."

While reassuring patients, many who asked each day about what would happen, we watched as the days passed and still no doctor had applied for the position.

My own children expressed confusion, too. Jack, my oldest and soon to be teenager, said, "Ah, Mom, come on, don't quit. You're home enough already."

"No, Mom, don't do it," said compassionate Benjamin. "If you quit, your patients won't have a mom or a doctor. We already have both. Don't do it, Mom."

"Well, if you're going to stay home, can Debbie, our sitter, be our second mom?" little Gray said, jumping rope around the kitchen.

My husband was happy for the family, eager to have me home full-time. He gave me a necklace with a golden angel pendant.

"An angel at rest," he said. "A long overdue rest."

The search team placed ads in psychiatric journals and national newspapers. My concerns of not locating a replacement were well founded as no applications were received.

I continued working with *The Artist's Way* by Julia Cameron and kept up my journaling. I was seeking another way to heal, one that would protect my mental health. Fearing the future, I wondered how would I function as a full-time mom? How would my patients fare without a psychiatrist?

Even as I hesitated, I knew I had to leave to save myself.

TIDAL WAVE

The waves of the sea help me get back to me.
—Surfer Today

THAT DECEMBER, ONE MONTH AFTER ANNOUNCING my resignation, I had a dream. In the vision, I was sitting on the porch of a lovely beach house, rocking with my daughter. We were drinking lemonade and enjoying the sights and sounds of the ocean. Suddenly, Gray looked up, worried.

"Mom, here comes a tidal wave."

"Oh, we will be fine," I said. "Let's stay. No need to run. We're safe."

So we sat as that wave washed over. Afterwards, the beach was clean and we were dry and happy. All the other houses were demolished, but ours was intact. There was a small convenience store open across the street. We walked over and purchased food and an alligator float after asking the owner, "Didn't that tidal wave hit you? How are you open?"

He smiled. "Oh, we're The Glorious Ascension at the Five and Dime. Welcome."

Well, that's a mystery.

We ran to play on the pristine beach.

And the next night, it began—the songs came. I woke at 5:05 a.m., and the writing started. *I Sing a Song for the Abused Child, the Song No One Wants to Hear* were the first words, but many followed. Lyrics poured out like water, filling my journal. One song followed another, as the dam burst, script overflowing. I was writing about events as far back as my student years, and as recent as the day before. Usually, I was home and wrote on the computer. If I was away from home, I wrote in a journal I carried with me everywhere.

It wasn't until I had printed and read them that I fully remembered the details of each story. One such lost memory was the murdering father and the dead-on-arrival baby, forgotten after third-year medical school until I pulled the paper off the printer and spoke the words out loud. I typed so furiously it was frightening, and I wondered if perhaps I had prayed too hard. How could I write about things I didn't consciously remember? How could I expect others to read and process such tragedies? But the course had been set. I was creating non-stop, recording the stories I had heard for the past ten years.

Alex was so relieved when I announced my resignation. But he would not have been happy if he'd known how the dirty clothes would pile up. I'm positive that he would not have rejoiced if he had known that in three short months he'd be doing his own laundry. The hypergraphia continued for months, but gradually tapered off so I could function. Cooking, washing clothes, and organizing schedules regained priority, but everyone, including me, would wish that I had not replaced the sitter.

SURRENDER

Let him lead me to the banquet hall,
and let his banner over me be love.
—Song of Solomon 2:4

I COULD HEAR GOD'S VOICE NOW. It was rumbling non-stop like a freight train, and I was transcribing as fast as I could. After this song "Surrender" was written, I discovered that as waterfowl, swans symbolize motherhood, love, and devotion, and that their connection with water represents creativity, intuition, dreaming, and emotions. As swans connect to earth, air, and sun, they create balance, exuding love, light, and all that is good.

Certainly, I was experiencing dreamy depths as I sought to balance out the years of listening. I was connecting to God as he whispered in my ear, giving way to the musical sway. The swan, a mystical icon of divine revelation, represented the beauty, passion, and protection I was craving. When I irreversibly surrendered, I was reborn. And although it would be years before grace abounded in my life, this creativity was a precursor to my heart opening and healing.

They say he transformed himself
into a beautiful bird,
then grabbed her by the nape.

Naked, he entered, feathers flying
in the heat of the motion, the movement.

Rocking in her bosom, cradled, seeking comfort
that only a lonely god craves.

Rending the veil, the maidenhead blossomed
as spirit fluttered on wings, hovered,
and then fully penetrated the virgin.

They say that Zeus transformed himself.
By Jove, I know he did, it's true,
because after he turned to swan,
he transformed Leda, too.

They say we stood by the pond,
beholding both the seduction
and the transformation,
yet still could not believe our eyes,
blinded by the splendor of their love.

That is what they say.

Odd things happened as the writing began. For weeks, my watch stopped at 5:05 a.m., documenting the moment I crept into my closet and wrote "I Sing a Song"—replacing the battery did not correct the time displayed. A bright, red rose bloomed in our garden, looming high over the snowbanks, causing my skeptical husband to ask if I had seen it.

"No," was my answer, as I furiously typed another song.

I finally looked at the flower encased in the ice of deep winter. I posed by the rose, and the photo he took is a treasured belonging.

A snowy owl sat for three days in the tree by our kitchen window. Momma pointed the owl out as I was too consumed to be bothered. With her prompting, reluctantly, I looked and saw a beautiful white owl staring back.

These events led me to recall a visitation from an angel choir earlier that August. Restless and not able to sleep, I came downstairs for a drink of water and was intent on checking the

Suburban once more for boogie boards, suitcases, and beach paraphernalia, as we were heading south first thing in the morning. Exhausted from life, work, and motherhood, I was looking forward to time with my parents and children on the North Carolina shore.

As I filled my glass, I gazed out into the yard. There in my garden were life-sized sparklers dazzling, at least forty different holy beings standing in what appeared to be a choral formation. One "angel," the largest, grandest, and brightest, stood in front, directing the others, her lit arms conducting her choir. Perhaps the most beautiful sight I had ever witnessed. But instead of going outside to join the dancing and singing, I ignored them and trudged back to bed, convinced that their presence had nothing to do with me. I was that damaged, that broken.

Sure that I could not find redemption with an angel chorus, I turned my back on them. It wasn't until the writing erupted that I even remembered the vision and realized they were a foreshadowing, a gift I had rejected.

MEL

Sexual abuse is not just abuse. It's sexual seduction of the individual and the family. It's a scourge on humanity. And it's happening right now in families, in churches and schools, and sports teams everywhere.

—Oprah Winfrey

"Dr. Burns, do you have a minute?"

I was packing my belongings, ready to head home, when I heard a tentative knock on the door. Fearing another emergency, a bobby pin slash, or a battery swallowed, I looked up hesitantly.

"Can I help you?"

It was Mel, our kitchen manager and cook. "Yes, Dr. Burns. Do you have a minute?"

"Of course, I do for you, Mel." I ushered him into my office.

Tentatively, he began his story. As the middle child of three, he was frequently in charge of his siblings. His older brother bullied him and often left the home when he should have been babysitting. Both his parents were alcoholics.

"I began remembering when I started working at the residential treatment facility," he said. "I thought cooking and meal planning were my jobs, but I was called to help with supervision, especially on weekends. Sometimes I was needed to monitor a wing while staff were involved in a therapeutic hold."

As a result, he became involved in the therapeutic milieu. Hoping to enhance the dining hall experience, he requested access to patients' medical records. Madeline and I agreed that Mel could review charts. However, he never told us how his flashbacks, migraines, alcoholism, diabetes, and post-traumatic stress disorder plagued him.

"I thought knowing the residents' psychiatric histories would improve my ability to care for them, in and out of the kitchen, Dr. Burns. But that's when their stories merged with mine. I began to remember my uncle's sexual assaults, and also understood how my parent's neglect and drinking affected me. You know, I was sober for years before coming to work here. Sometimes it seemed being sober made the flashbacks and mood swings more frequent. It was only in reviewing the histories of these patients that I began to put it all together—the puzzle of my childhood."

Working with the clinical staff inspired Mel to get to the bottom of his story. As Mel's dreams and memories became vivid, understanding the role that neglect and sexual abuse had played in his life was his goal. If not, he was certain it would forever haunt him. His uncle, a frequent babysitter, sexually molested him.

"I remember nights standing by the window with my younger brother, staring into the darkness, looking for my parents. We waited late into the night, frightened and hungry, falling asleep huddled together on the floor. The reason I'm such a good cook is that I learned early, feeding my brothers." Tears rolled down his face as he spoke.

In his dreams, Mel saw the two-story house where he was raised burn to the ground, with his uncle in it. He knew he was angry, but couldn't feel anything. So he visited his home and the cemetery where his family was buried. He sought release from the diseases that defined his life—obesity, hypertension, diabetes, migraines, and knee pain—and from the emotional numbing, hyper-vigilance, panic attacks, and social isolation from post-traumatic stress disorder. Weeping silently as he recited these memories, the relief he felt lay between us. Since going to visit his home and the cemetery, his headaches had improved and his blood sugar was more stable. He was kinder to himself, taking time to eat regularly. Although sad, he was also joyous.

"I don't know what would have happened to me if I hadn't worked here with you, Madeline, and the children. I am so grateful. Please, Dr. Burns, write my story. Speak about this whenever you present on childhood trauma. I want folks to know how I remembered, to learn how my headaches improved with remembering, to demonstrate how I learned to love myself. Sobriety set me free and created a healing, but my work here has given me the key to unlock a door that was shut tight. You were such a part of that, Dr. Burns. Thank you. I am going to miss you, and so are the children."

"I will miss you, Mel. My love and respect for you has been great, but now it is boundless."

We hugged and said goodnight, promising to stay in touch after I left.

I called my husband. "I'm late. Start homework and supper. I'm on my way."

Once more, I witnessed the toll that neglect and abuse takes on a child, on the life of that child grown up. But this time I had a tool, a way to make things different.

I sat at my computer and wrote what Mel had just told me, the song that would tell his tale—not of a victim, but of a strong, lionhearted fellow who wasn't afraid to face his past because he knew that in knowing and naming his abusers, he was liberating himself.

Months later, I called him. "Mel, your story is one of the first paintings in my *Black and White and Red All Over* series. You're going to be a star!"

We laughed together.

"What is that, Dr. Burns? Black, white, and red?"

"Paintings. I make linen panels, forty-by-fifty-two inches, Gray's height. I paint each one black, then white, then red. The colors reflect my belief that child abuse is black and white in plain sight, yet ignored. Red symbolizes the blood spilling over this epidemic because of our apathy, and the frayed edges depict the tattered and uneven nature of life. Then I place pieces of tissue paper, collaging an image that keeps repeating, similar to abuse."

"Oh, Dr. Burns, that sounds amazing. I want one."

"Of course. Come by and we'll create yours in the studio together."

And we did.

He remembers now what it was like back then.

*Dreams and memories press, suffocating,
drawing out his breath.*

*He panics when alone, awakening
to an abandoned house not filled with love.
Table empty, no mother, no father.*

*He remembers now, the scary hours
when he watched over them all,
when he was only four.*

*Standing by the dark, dirty window,
waiting alone, looking for parents
who never came, who were never on time.*

*Sober watching,
waiting for someone to come and care.*

Remembers now what it was like back then.

*Black gaps filling in as the angels sing the story
that crashes in his head.*

*Dark red pain, scary tremors,
depths untouched before by his brain
—memories scrunched tight, hiding in his body,
not to be heard, felt, or seen.*

JULIA W. BURNS

"God, no, I am not going to do this.
Not going to remember it.
What it was like back then."

Flames and water roll into his dreams,
chased by men in a fiery furnace
which even hell has not seen.

God bless this child, quaking in fear,
abandoned to his uncle's evil urges.

God bless him in his struggle to be free.

Unearth memories, drive to strange places,
looking for clues.

Red houses and ghostly cemeteries
haunt his search.

He remembers now what it was like back then.
Remembers so his headaches will disappear.
He fills his journal with darkness
as his heart lightens with peace.

DAVE MATTHEWS

His heart full of love, love, love.
Love, love, love.
Love, love was all around
— Dave Matthews

RAY, A CHILDCARE WORKER, HAD WRITTEN to the musician, Dave Matthews, asking if he would play for our residents.

> Dear Dave,
> I'm writing to ask if you could come to White Pines, a treatment facility for emotionally disturbed children and adolescents, and play for us while you are in Durham. I've been a fan forever. It would mean so much.

He included letters from the residents, with pictures they had drawn and their requests to hear him sing. Dave was touring with Tim Reynolds on an unplugged tour and agreed to play for our small audience of fifty in the downtown Stanley Auditorium. A private concert for White Pines was arranged.

"No, Dr. Burns, I'm not going," Joe said. "I don't like Dave Matthews."

"What? Joe, have you heard "A Christmas Song"? Listened to "Ants Marching"? Ridiculous. Come on, you're riding with me.

If you don't like it, I'll have someone bring you back to campus. I promise."

"OK, Dr. Burns, I'll come. But I like Metallica. Dave Matthews is boring."

Debbie, our sitter, brought my children. Jack asked a friend, Michael, to come along. We had told him that Jack had a violin concert because we were sworn to secrecy. Michael started trembling in the lobby when he heard Dave Matthews playing. I thought he was going to faint.

A new childcare worker acting as security tried to stop us as we walked in. "No one can come in who doesn't work at White Pines."

I hoped he wouldn't send the children away, and I was trying to persuade him when Ray walked up and said, "Let them in. Geez, Barry, that's Dr. Burns and it's her birthday. Let her go."

And with that, the "bouncer" stepped aside and the music commenced. Dancing in the aisles with Joe, Johnny, Jim, and Sandra during an acoustic rendition of *A Christmas Song* was otherworldly.

Michael continued to shake, and it took us a long time to come off the cloud—the happiness, the thrill, lasted for days. Divinity had spirited itself inside and outside of us through those melodic refrains, lifting fear, even if just for a few hours.

After the concert, I only had a few days, and they went quickly. The three-month notice ended, and still no psychiatrist had applied.

GOING AWAY

And then a river of tears.
Much clinging to Paul, not wanting to let him go.
They knew they would never see him again—he
had told them quite plainly. The pain cut deep.
Then, bravely, they walked him down to the ship.
—Acts 20:37-38

"Dr. Burns, we're celebrating your departure. The kids want their own event so they can read the stories and poems they wrote. Nothing sad, I promise."

Mel was planning two parties. Saying goodbye might last for an eternity.

As we listened to each other, my patients and I ate cake, reveling in our relationship. It was bittersweet, but lovely. Patty's tulip painting hangs in my studio. A scrapbook of our time at White Pines—playing pool, eating pizza, and dancing in the aisles—holds our memories.

When the last day ended, I turned in my keys, walked out the door, and drove away from my colleagues, patients, and professional life—with great apprehension. My identity was in defending the abused child. What song would I sing if I were no longer medical director, prescriber, and treatment-team consultant? What would it be like taking care of my children and being home full-time?

"Where are you going?"

I am away. I am leaving you behind.

"Where are you going?"

*Under the sea in search of a red thread
to replace the black stone that sits in my chest,
where my heart used to be.*

"Why are you leaving?"

*I am leaving to find another,
one who has become lost.*

"Why are you leaving?"

*I am leaving because no matter where I turn,
this space no longer contains my body.*

"When will we see you?"

*At night, when the moon is red
and the werewolves rip flesh with bloody teeth.*

"When will we see you?"

*At daytime, when the sun is white and the incubus
sleeps in a cave, away from my children.*

"How will we know you?"

*You will know I am gone as a vapor rises over the
garden. Red roses growing in the center will give
pure perfume.*

"Who will check my heartbeat?"

*There will be a white coat, steel-cold stethoscope
with a bell to listen for the beat.*

"Who will check my heartbeat?"

*I will turn my ear toward the wind and listen to
know if you are still beating.*

"Who will hear our stories?"

The angels will hear, the wind will tell, and the water will wash over for healing.

"Who will hear our stories?"

The ones with the red thread wrapped around their hearts, beating in the center of the small black stone, will listen and learn from you, as I have.

"Who will hold our grief?"

The wailing of the angels will resound around the orb, but will never hold your grief.

"Who will hold our grief?"

The weeping of the wind blowing wildly through the meadow will search for the mountain, but even that cannot contain our anguish.

"Where are you going?"

I am diving under the sea. I am going to tell the mermaids.

WISDOM

*I know why the caged bird sings.
It's one of the greatest gifts you can give yourself,
to forgive.
Forgive everybody.*

—Maya Angelou

MY FIRST ATTEMPT AT HEALING was to keep writing while hunkered down, protecting myself, not reflecting on the wounds. Years as a therapist told me this wouldn't work, but human nature seductively coaxed me into ignoring the pain. Fervently hoping that when spring arrived, I would thaw and blossom with the apple trees, I prayed for wholeness even as I was confused about what was broken. Scared that peace would never come, I rambled through an apple orchard, searching for meaning in the flowering and rebirth.

*Wisdom lives in trees
growing in rows in an orchard,
black bones bared to weather—*
January's mercury did not rise above zero.
*These were living trees,
beckoning villagers to be still, to become one,
as roots, her stick-like fingers,
cling deeply to a stone-cold ground,*

and her arms beg the sky,
rock me waxing moon.

Charred wings lift white and gray clouds
as ice crystals fall,
frozen sculptures mirroring skeletal ribbons.

Black rhythm bangs out white,
ridden by winter's rage.

These trees live in an orchard by a road
outside our village green and fountain,
where a copper girl stands erect.

Her arms arise, branches ever bearing buds,
suspended capsules slumbering,
awaiting rugged, higher light for birth.

Some jesters believe they are mortal, but not so,
for the immersed know of miracles
—nectar, apple crisp, and dumplings,
the humming buzz, the seasonal ring.

Boughs embalmed in a frozen field
just beyond a winding asphalt trail.

Leave Eve with the apple's core.
Hear the wailing, beckoning us to sweep our limbs into
the harsh freeze
and grow as the apple tree does.

Hard cores, wooden layers,
wrap diminishing, concentric waves.

Live with winter's fleeting caresses,
bones bared to seasonal tides.

I knew that more listening—and especially more believing—for me, was not healthy. In my war against abuse, compassion not condemnation, love not judgment, and prayer not complaining were needed. Yet I had appointed myself judge and jury. Everyone was guilty—the perpetrators, social workers, case workers, administrators, parents, and childcare workers. No one seemed committed to naming and preventing child abuse, and in my pride and bitterness, I failed to look up and see love and healing.

Fortunately, my children adored me and showed it daily. Their hugs and endless requests for rides to soccer and school kept me distracted.

"Duck, Mom, duck," Benjamin would shout, as soon as we rolled into the school parking lot.

"I can't, Benjamin. I'm driving," I would reply.

Teaching all three to play the violin through the Suzuki method was challenging, but a stimulating distraction. Our daily practice sessions, although sometimes conflictual, connected us to our love of each other and music. It appeared that both violin and singing songs were paths to wholeness. I began to mend without a diagnosis. My breathing normalized. I stayed home, immersing myself in the mundane yet exquisite dance of motherhood.

But I'd had little comprehension of just how demanding life as a stay-at-home mom could be. I loved cooking, although the menu choices were limited—was it pizza or spaghetti tonight? Playing whiffle ball with the children, breaking up arguments, washing skinned knees, all gave me joy, but keeping track of the household chores was onerous.

I was much better at interviewing patients and writing prescriptions, and I missed my team and patients. I missed myself. Keeping up with everyone's schedules was proving impossible. Laundry was never-ending, and helping with homework was laborious. Often, Gray wanted me to sit beside her while she studied.

We were disagreeing about something this one afternoon, and I said, "Look, you can do this by yourself. Call me if you need help. I don't like sitting beside you while you do homework."

"Well, if you don't like helping with homework," she said, "why did you quit work?"

Good question. I headed down the basement stairs, with another load of laundry.

One day, I was stuffing another load of dirty clothes into the washer when Jack came down the stairs and said, "Hey, Mom, would you give me ten dollars a week if I did laundry?"

Wanting to do cartwheels on the basement floor, I casually turned around. "What?"

"Could I do laundry, Benjamin's and mine, for ten dollars a week?"

"Sure," I agreed, nonchalantly.

Later, he tried to take it back when he realized how much work it was, but it was too late. The bargain had been struck. We increased his allowance, but he earned far more than we ever paid him.

A few months later, Jack walked down the basement stairs again. This time, we were both doing laundry.

"Mom, I'm worried about Benjamin. He's only had one pair of dirty underwear this week."

Not knowing how to respond, but knowing what he said was likely true, I honored his concern with a commitment to speak to his brother.

That talk went something like, "If you want your brother to keep doing your laundry, you better change underpants every day. We can't have him worrying, and you don't want to go to school dirty."

I'm not sure if it worked. I never asked. But I did keep a closer eye at bath time.

INNOCENT LOVE

The course of true love never did run smooth.
—William Shakespeare

ONE DAY, MOMMA AND I WERE SHOPPING with all three children, having decided that a trip to the grocer was better than starvation. We were standing in the checkout line waiting our turn for the cashier when Gray turned to me and said, "Mom, what's s-e-x? What's sexing?"

Wondering why we were having this conversation now—in front of Momma, our neighbor standing behind us, and the cashier waiting in front—I turned to her and said, "Sex? What is sex?"

The boys were doubled over, but Gray was serious.

"Yes. What is that?"

Gray had noticed a shiny brightly colored magazine cover touting, "14 Ways to Have an Orgasm or Help All Your Boyfriends Have One Too."

Gee whiz, I never knew it was so complicated and that we needed twelve magazines with fourteen new techniques to find your man and keep him happy. Teen love. Learn to Say, I Love You in Three Languages. How to Know If You're Really Ready to Go All The Way. Seven Sure Ways to Lush Your Lips and Capture Your Love. Body Boosting Tips to Make

Sure You're Never Alone, Flirting Floozies. How To Make Sure You Are The One. Love Chat Tells All. What's His Love Style? What's Yours? Teenlove.com. Whoa, I'm in Love. Eight Habits to Ruin Romance. Hot Date Beauty Guide. Who Kisses and Tells and Who doesn't—Find Out Here. Quiz #1: Will Your Love Last? A Good Boyfriend Would Be Smart Not to Try to Make Me Feel Dumb!

Standing at the checkout with my bologna, cheese, chicken, and bread, and with my momma, daughter, and two sons is not when I want to read fourteen ways to come. I don't want them to read it, either. Ever. Questions and quizzes for the young and restless to answer, but not when I'm trying to checkout, please.

Benjamin saved the day by informing Gray that he knew about sex, and if she needed to know something to ask him.

"Don't ask Mom, for Pete's sake, Gray. Ask somebody who knows."

When we got home, I got out the book we bought for the boys about body parts belonging to me and only me, and this is how God created you.

"You are beautiful, and your body is a temple," I told Gray. "It is yours and yours only."

That autumn, I sat at our breakfast table, spellbound by the beauty of Gray jumping and flipping on the trampoline with her friend Jenny as an early snowfall surrounded them.

*Standing at the kitchen window,
just after our first snowstorm,
I was watching as the blue broke through the gray.*

*Looking out, I saw my daughter jumping,
jumping with a friend.*

*The sun bouncing on the trampoline
as the canvas shoved them, pushing back.*

Jumping because they could,
in a white storm or the blue.

Staring, I could not move, so rooted was I
to this place of being eight again.

They sat side by side
on the roof of her playhouse,
sharing stories, heads bent,
coupling to whisper secrets,
so close, each ear caught the murmurs.

Oranges match their soccer shorts,
treetops echo yellow socks.

When they bit into their apples,
we could taste the tang
pulling with every mouthful,
savoring it.

Touch their laughter rolling off that roof.

And so I stood still,
placing this space and this moment
in our lives.

Light shimmering abounds our seeing
through the window and beyond.

Remember the reddening leaves
as snow brings freeze.

But for now, we blaze like coloring trees
in this palette in birdsong;
this jumping in the stillness.

    The children's meltdowns and their hugs, the way we were living together, convinced me that I was headed in the right direction. Surely it would be enough.

    But that spring, after returning home from a visit to my parents, I looked around our messy den and felt overwhelmed. The room, completely clean upon my arrival home two days ago, was now a disaster. Resentment at being treated like a maid welled up.

> *Candy wrappers that had been thrown away*
> *in my absence, now littered the room.*
> *Cans, trash, and dirty dishes piled up—not mine,*
> *but then not anyone else's either,*
> *because nobody made the mess*
> *that no one was cleaning*
> *now that the maid had returned.*
> *This mess lit a fire inside me,*
> *along with a new contract for our life,*
> *that when no one leaves their dirty underwear*
> *for nobody to pick up,*
> *it will lay there, forever soiled.*
> *The maid didn't come home*
> *from vacation this year,*
> *but the musical doctor did*
> *and kicked out no one,*
> *nobody, and the maid.*
> *Without the quicker picker-upper,*
> *we are all better off.*

It was much easier to do my children's chores than to remind them to do them. Nagging and posting a chore chart on the refrigerator did not work. Often, we would check at the end of the week to find the chart empty. Arguments ensued about whose turn it was to do the dishes, and who had the most homework, or who hadn't practiced violin.

I had counseled depressed stay-at-home mothers that working outside the home is nine-to-five, while working inside the home is twenty-four-seven. I was living that truth and singing that song over and over.

PATSY

Friends come and friends go,
but a true friend sticks by you like family.
—Proverbs 18:24

PATSY, A GARDENER, AND I MET IN EARLY FALL when I hired her to recreate a lily garden by the driveway. We were planting together when she looked down.

"What's your job? What do you do?"

"I am the medical director of an eighteen-bed psychiatric hospital for children and adolescents, and I manage medications for hundreds more."

Her succinct response: "You need to quit."

Patsy saw my suffering, and by calling it out boldly, she inspired me. Others called it seasonal depression, homesickness, being overwhelmed with work and motherhood, but she named it correctly: burnout. She understood that the stories demanded digestion, and as that required intention, she coaxed me to live slowly.

"A death has occurred, and you are in mourning," she said. "This work is hurting you. Paint, it will revive you. Listen to yourself."

She recommended that I read *The Artist's Way* by Julia Cameron. And I did. So if God gets first place for jumpstarting my creative career, Patsy was his earthly angel. She took my dried, barren soul, set it ablaze, and stood back watching as visions, dreams, and songs burst forth.

It took many months of retirement before I recognized the extent of the numbness and grief as Patsy and I painted, gardened, and wrote together. She was balm to my soul.

The conversation with God was ongoing. Awakening early to pore over the Bible, I searched for meaning and the message that would set me free. Struggling even as the writing and painting pressed forward, I urgently transcribed messages, poems, and songs that sprang fully formed. My hope was in the songs now that I had quit working. I had to write, submit to publishers, and pray. Write, submit, and pray, waiting for the day that the news would spread about the epidemic of child abuse. Hadn't I promised to tell the mermaids?

Few of my friends and family knew of my suffering. They simply thought I was taking a break from doctoring to be Mom. Even Alex didn't realize the deep wounds because I stayed silent. In part, I didn't tell because I didn't understand. Also, I kept it a secret because I was ashamed, thinking something was terribly wrong if I couldn't work and take care of my patients.

Patsy and I saw each other frequently. We created music, frolicked in the snow, or cross country skied. I started taking cello lessons and playing the piano again. Resigning had been unthinkable until her insight unlocked something. The resonance I felt with her declaration was so profound that I handed in my resignation days after we met. Her friendship sustained me, until one cold, wet spring day—a day when you fervently wish for the sun's warmth, but instead grab your long underwear to insulate from the freeze. Patsy invited me to paint, which we usually did in her heated but drafty, garage. When I got to her house, she showed me a beautiful angel she had started. She helped me gather my colors, gold and purple, then said she needed to run some errands.

"I'll go with you." I was surprised that she would invite me over and leave.

But she looked at me and shook her head. "I won't be long. You stay here and paint. Don's coming by."

Something was odd. She left and didn't come back for a long while.

She had frequently said, *"You've heard enough. You need to stop."* But despite this, she had another story for me.

"I'd like to tell you something," said Don, her handyman. "Patsy thinks it's a good idea. Is that okay?" And in monotone, he recited his story.

He told of the life that he and his brother had shared with a violent father and a depressed, passive mother.

"Both my parents came from broken homes. My mother was sexually abused by her father. My father was abandoned at the age of three by an alcoholic, abusive father. A string of my mother's violent boyfriends followed. My parent's marriage was also violent. They didn't know how to take care of themselves or us."

*Don was sweeping and I was painting,
coloring in the lines of the angels who started that
glorious ascension to the five and dime.*

*You can purchase the goods there
if you travel the distance.
The store lives next door.*

*When he told me another story,
this time about brooms, circles, brains,
and mothers who fall out and around themselves,
forgetting they need to sweep up the remains left
behind when death comes, the physical ends, and
it's over.*

*Sweeping the studio, he started
and finished the story.*

*Raising dust in the air as I tried to continue
ascending, purple and blue mixing,
an inferior rendition of the flight
the angels are taking without us.*

*We painted, swept, and circled
as the story of his life continued
—coming home from school one day,
his father told the boys to go to the basement
to sweep up the dog's leftover dinner:*

*"It's smelling up the air and the room
and this house and our life."*

*So the brothers descend the staircase,
steep, dark, and dingy the lie they believe
as they struggle and bicker over who is to sweep
and who is to hold the dust bin.*

Gather up the leftovers of their mother.

*In order to avoid the beating
waiting for them upstairs, they swept
those remains, with the trash of their lives,
in the garbage.*

*He swept as he talked. Swept, not wept,
making little circles of dust that rose in the air.*

*I painted the angels that were guarding him,
outlined clearly in the circles of the broom.
Sweeping the room clean, throwing out the
leftovers, and trying to save the remains.*

Don, homeless and addicted, was unable to work. Without Patsy's intervention, he would have no friends, food, or money. After five months of painting and creating with Patsy, I was bitterly disappointed that our sanctuary had been violated. Angry that I had found a friend who would absolve me of the responsibility of listening, then arrange one more story. I marveled at her callousness. I realized she was trying to save him, but I had little to give and much to lose in becoming involved in his life. I was alone and totally absorbed in my brokenness.

After suffering so many losses, with this last insult my separation from God deepened. I had no hope and felt like a hypocrite—my soul did not rejoice, even as I continued to teach Sunday School, go to church, sing in the choir, and lead a lay Eucharistic ministry, taking communion to shut-ins. In my stubbornness, I blamed God for the stories I heard and the suffering I experienced. I couldn't find forgiveness for either of us, but it was myself I blamed the most. I had known God intimately all my life, yet now, in this betrayal by my friend, I felt forsaken.

Utterly displaced and homesick for him, I pined for what was easily within reach. My judgement of others was so deep only blackness existed, and I wept in silence, creating a place of hurt so shut off that I could not experience love, God's or anyone else's.

How my husband stood by me, I do not know, except that he truly lived up to our marriage vows, *for better or worse.*

REDEMPTION

I have swept away your offenses like a cloud,
your sins like the morning mist.
Return to me, for I have redeemed you.
—Isaiah 44:22 NIV

HUMBLING MYSELF, I PLEADED FOR GOD'S TOUCH and grace, gradually allowing light to penetrate every dark place. Slowly and painstakingly, after much meditation, prayer, and spiritual direction, I began to understand that people—not God—were abusing my patients. As my feelings vacillated between anger and numbness, I began to realize that the Holy Spirit hovered over each abused patient, viewing the beating terror and weeping with the victims.

Finally, I was able to let God off the hook. I realized that my patients' wounds dictated their lives because their abuse wasn't remembered and integrated. Invisible hurts continued to surface in surprising ways as the cycle of abuse continued. The same would be true for me if I could not remember, lament, mourn, and forgive.

And so thousands of songs were sung that first year—songs exposing the invisible. Through prayer, writing, painting, and deep searching, I gradually accepted that perpetrators were once small abused children, too. During their abuse, neurological traces formed, and as these wounded children grew, they forced sexual experiences on another generation of children, searching for a familiar connection. And as serial child molesters raped children, caretakers turned their heads, living their own scripts from childhood, unable or unwilling to notice, refusing to intervene, enabling darkness. So many humans deny trauma because of their own particular wounds of witnessing abuse without the power to enable change.

Finally, I accepted the truth: God did not abuse my patients, and most of the time the perpetrators were abused first.

MIRANDA

*The saddest thing about betrayal
is that it never comes from your enemies.*
                              —Anonymous

THE FOLLOWING FALL, APPLES FILLED OUR ORCHARDS. Trees yielded, in a spectacular display of green and red, lovely fruit for our table. This blossoming was in stark contrast to the front-page news of a sixteen-year-old mildly mentally handicapped girl, Miranda, who was fatally stabbed in a crack house. Her boyfriend was arrested for the crime. Miranda, resident of institutions for years, began prostituting and using drugs immediately upon her discharge.

Years earlier, I met Miranda on a bright spring day. The shining sun was gradually melting layers of snow that had covered the ground for months.

"Ah, Dr. Burns, don't you smell it? Skunk—a sure sign of spring!" Miranda's caseworker said, as we walked in from the parking lot of the state psychiatric hospital.

The chief of psychiatry had called for a consultation, hoping that I might be able to assist with diagnosis and treatment.

"Sure, I smell it. Who could miss it? But I prefer the smell of honeysuckle to skunk."

A brooding, troubled thirteen-year-old child, Miranda looked much older than her age. Initially guarded and belligerent, she quickly transformed into a friendly, cooperative patient. Abused by her mother, father, and various relatives, she trusted no one. Her jet-black hair covered several piercings. She presented with a goth look—, dark black eyeshadow and thick mascara obscured her lovely dark eyes. Her frightening appearance was an attempt to hide emotional distress.

The family did everything they could to undermine her sense of safety. One December, when Santa Claus visited the hospital, Miranda ran screaming to the time-out room. It took a while to uncover the root of her hysteria, but eventually she told a story of her father and uncles dressed as Santa, attacking and raping her. In this cruel act, they robbed her of an archetypal character representing kindness and giving, destroying the miracle and love of Christmas.

Miranda appeared sophisticated despite cognitive challenges, and this made her a frequent scapegoat. Often, she did not understand teasing, so relationships were unstable. Her academic function was poor because teachers did not fully comprehend the scope of her learning disorder. She had little ability to defend herself against sexual predators, having been groomed for sex since birth.

Home was a nightmare, and school offered little comfort. She performed what she knew best: sexual favors. The hospital treatment team decided to place Miranda at St. Anthony's, a residential center specializing in treating developmentally disabled girls. She started to improve and was able to organize her behavior. She began to do chores, take responsibility in the kitchen, and clean up after supper. Her ability to read and write improved.

However, about eight months into her residential stay at St. Anthony's, Miranda became increasingly angry and oppositional. She refused to leave school in the afternoon and was resistant to staff. Her hygiene was poor. She isolated herself, and her friendships deteriorated. A peer filed an incident report that Miranda was having a sexual relationship with a male nurse. The administrator who received the report discounted it because it was written by another resident, not a staff person. No one reported the information to her caseworker. The report was not reviewed by the Quality Assurance Committee. It was lost and forgotten.

Six months later, a staff person witnessed the same nurse having sex with Miranda. Another incident report was filed, and this time the Quality Assurance Committee reviewed the evidence and found the allegation to be true. The nurse was placed on probation and required to go to weekly supervision. Miranda was discharged to yet another facility. Thus, the victim was punished, losing her home and the relationships she had forged.

Not long after, we heard she was pregnant and living on the streets. We wondered if she would keep her baby and how they would live. Soon after, we heard Miranda had miscarried and was hooking for drugs, trying to find peace in a world that had shown her only hostility.

On the evening I learned about Miranda's death, I had gone to the orchard with my children. Apple pie was Benjamin's favorite, and he made the crust while I peeled and sliced apples. His life so different from hers, so filled with love and opportunities. So many doors were open for my children that had been slammed shut for my patients, and for their parents, shut even earlier.

> *Supper over, we washed our dishes,*
> *soaking the crystal*
> *to see if we could find our reflection.*
>
> *It was a ritual cleansing, washing away dirt*
> *like the dishwasher never could*
> *—washing and rinsing the sins from our feasting,*
> *standing as we were that night,*
> *on the back of her innocence.*
>
> *She was stabbed ten times in a tenement,*
> *living in hell, dying in that crack.*

Who held the knife that tore her body,
shredding her soul? Who will bear the tale of our
indifference to the molestations that have formed
her since her birth?

Let me find the mountain and climb to its heights,
a mountain so high it can smother this sadness.
Let me soar to the top,
where the lonely wolves howl.

And if I cannot ascend, then I must continue
this mad polishing, circling the cutlery
—pieces so tarnished they are almost black
and beyond recognition—rubbing in circles,
burnishing the darkness that is covering our souls,
seeking a brilliance we may never find,
as we rinse off the polish in scalding water.

Making a luster we hope will last forever,
we dry each piece.

Circling the stains on the silver,
rubbing out the blots with a white cloth
so a radiance emerges.

Rubbing and scrubbing to cover the choking
and heaving that I heard in my kitchen
with the reading of her story:
another of my children dying in a room,
lying there bleeding, all alone again.

What song were the angels singing while she lay
on the floor receiving that beating,
giving way to his knife?

Where were the angels hovering
in that covering of her truth?

Who else was hiding behind the polish?

What lies in the black and silver darkness
while her blood soaks our rags?

And in this shrouding, we must continue
our cleaning, polishing silver after supper
on a Sunday evening,
after the reading of her death.

As Alex finished the newspaper account, he said, "Hey Julia, the paper says that the girl who died in the crack house was in a residential hospital. Her name was Miranda. They think she died in a drug deal gone bad, stabbed to death. Do you know her?"

He knew by my sobs that I did.

LIMBO

Limbo is not a good place to be.
—Bill Joy

THE URGENCY I FELT TO PUBLISH was tremendous. My stories and songs appeared in a Buddhist journal, church publications, and magazines for sexual-abuse survivors. The rawness of my songs confused my audiences: "We can't publish this story unless you omit the details of the abuse. People will not be able to relate to your message," I heard frequently. "If you leave out the references to God and evil, you'll have an easier time publishing. Cull the religious, Julia. You'll get more interest."

My paintings hung in libraries and coffee shops; colleagues and friends encouraged me, but listeners were few. The worst part was waiting for weeks or months after a submission without hearing anything. Although I could heal myself by writing and painting, I needed an audience to create restoration for others. No editor stepped forward to create the definitive book of Dr. Burns's songs. And if that wasn't going to happen, then I was going to heal as a physician.

To work or not to work was the question. There was only one other child psychiatrist in town, and job offers were plentiful. After about eighteen months at home, I started considering some of them. I was torn. The years of training, mastering psychiatry, had been long and arduous. I wanted to find new patients—perhaps ones who weren't abused.

Michael, the CEO of Mental Health Connections, called frequently: "Dr. Burns, if you'll come work for us, you can set your schedule. If you prefer, you can leave at three so you'll be home with your children after school. You can do evaluations and keep the patients you find interesting, and refer the others to outside therapists. We need you and want you to come. Please let us know."

So I started seeing patients again. I didn't know what else to do; at forty-three years old, I had trained to be a doctor until age thirty-five. It seemed reasonable, and this time it was different. Completing initial psychiatric evaluations and prescribing medications were my primary responsibilities. I did not do any therapy, and thought my limited contact with patients would protect me. Participation at treatment-team meetings was not required unless the patient was doing poorly. Because I referred sexual trauma to other providers, I completed two new psychiatric evaluations a day, with added medication checks. The primary caseworkers attended all patient interviews, and if they were absent, we rescheduled. My nurse manager, Jean, was terrific, checking weights and vital signs, doing nutritional counseling and family psychoeducation, managing my schedule without ever double-booking me.

At first, going back to work seemed right, as I felt confident and capable in my old role. The caseworkers were empowered when we worked on difficult cases together. Everything would be fine until I heard another abuse story or witnessed a mother telling her daughter, "Liar. Your daddy did not do that! You little lying bitch, shut up."

Or Ryan, a young boy, describing his multiple personalities: "They live inside this place that has computers, and they live inside my mind. They like to stay in me because they want to do me first. I don't know why. They don't like to be outside, because they like the people of the mind." By drawing "the people of the mind" together, coaxing them outside, he gained mastery over them.

"Dr. Burns, do you have a pill that makes bad men go away? I'm afraid to go to sleep. I'm afraid I will die."

Yes, I have a pill that will help you sleep, and I'm afraid to sleep, too. Afraid if I do, you will die. Worried if I don't create the best treatment plan, you will remain in your home where they are hurting you. Yes, let me prescribe the pill to make it better so neither one of us dies.

I would then retreat and ask the primary therapist to come and take the child for a session. After finishing another evaluation, I would go home and write a song, this time about little boys and computers of the mind, and girls who lie about their daddies. And I would try to find a place to sing it.

"Hey, Alex," I said, "I think we were right. Part-time employment seems to be good. I have time to make all the soccer games and violin concerts. So far, I haven't taken one sexually abused child onto my caseload. I'm happier being with the children now that I'm not home all the time. I don't miss doing laundry, and I love my patients."

I was enthusiastic about my work at Mental Health Connections. The children enjoyed their new sitter and coming home to a "Mom-free" zone. The songs kept coming. My research on PTSD continued, although I still didn't know I had it.

Reminding myself of the war veteran who volunteers for three tours of duty, I refused to retire. I'm not sure if I returned because it was all I knew and I was good at it, or if I had to prove that it hadn't beaten me. Still, I was unable to obtain treatment for burnout and secondary PTSD because the disorder remained virtually unknown. Burnout was recognized in physicians, but little was being done for it. Secondary PTSD was nameless.

NINE-ELEVEN

*The Lord is my shepherd
as a man holds a box-cutter.
I shall not want,
and a woman phones her husband.
He makes me to lie down
as a jet crashes
in green pastures.
He leads me beside
the fiery gates of steel and
the still waters. He restores my soul
as a priest administers the last rites.*

He leads me in the paths of righteousness
to a fireman. They die in each other's arms
for his name's sake. Yea, though I walk
by two hundred twenty crumbling stories,
through the valley of the shadow,
a cardinal sings of death.

*As a blue jay chases the red one away,
I will fear—he is hungrier—
no evil.
He is bigger.
Thy rod and thy staff, they comfort,
and a cardinal sings to me.*

Water circles a pond as
thou preparest a table
where one hundred fish swim
in the presence,
and this flowing creates the breath
of my enemies.

As fish breathe under water
and my cup runneth over,
once there were three.

He anoints my head with oil.
Now there are one hundred.

Surely goodness and mercy will follow.

Fish swim, fish breathe, and a cardinal sings to me
all the days of my life.

And I will dwell,
now the thousands search
in the house of the Lord,
for loved ones to say goodbye.

I'll miss you forever.

—Inspired by Psalm 23

SEPTEMBER 11, 2001. Perhaps the last to learn about the bombings of the World Trade Center towers, I had turned to writing as soon as the children left for school, after switching off the television, radio, and telephone. School starting meant more time for writing. The phone rang several times that morning, but I ignored it, continuing with my work: typing, editing, trying to create something that a publisher would print so the world could sing along. I knew nothing about the danger or the suffering in New York City.

The weather channel warned that a hurricane was projected to hit the island where our beach house stood. We had traded six feet of snow in the winter for a house on a barrier island in the summer, and I was praying that it would not be demolished. It was a selfish prayer, and when I heard about the World Trade Center towers, I made a pact with God never to be consumed about a storm destroying my beach house. I have kept that promise.

Late afternoon, I turned off the computer and listened to the answering machine: "Julia, this is Momma. I know you are praying, but I want you to call me and let me know how you are. Doesn't David, Alex's good friend from college work near the World Trade buildings that blew up? Have you heard from him? I'm praying. I know you're praying, too. Call. I need to hear your voice."

I ran from the phone to the television in disbelief, only to have her words confirmed. The TV showed the tallest, most powerful towers in the world crumble and melt into ash. Stunned, I quickly converted my prayers for good weather at the beach to safety for those in New York. The children came home from school frightened because they had watched those images of destruction in their classrooms and wanted to know how our New York friends were. I couldn't tell them because I didn't know.

There was a pall over our village as this dark disaster hung over us. Silence ruled, and in an attempt to process the tragedy, I sat by my pond, writing. Fish swam and birds fought by the feeder even though there was enough food. Their struggle for dominance reminded me of the fear that killed the thousands in New York. The fight over something not visible, not seen. Division creating scarcity in the kingdom of God's plenty.

Our family was preparing to visit a friend who was recovering from brain surgery. He'd collapsed from a seizure and was diagnosed with glioblastoma multiform. We felt compelled to see him, despite the recent bombings, because we didn't know how long he would live. We wanted to be together, and the terrorist attack only increased this desire. The devastating silent mourning which held everyone in its aftermath clung to me as I prepared the children's clothes for our trip to the city.

*Gray and black smoke still hung in the air
of our New City as we walked
toward the drug store.
Strolling down her sidewalks with my daughter,
I thought that our director had made a mistake,
that on this crackling fall day, dazzled by the sun,
maybe he had forgiven and forgotten
that Tuesday ever happened.*

*The day our towers of wealth
crumbled with our people wailing inside.*

"Mommy, I wish I were a dog.

*If I were Pumpkin,
I wouldn't have to know about today.*

*And tomorrow,
I wouldn't have to know about today, either."*

I wish I were a dog, too, honey.

*As we breathed in these black and gray ashes,
dust fell away to dust.*

*I wondered as the next exhalation
traveled from my spirit into this darkened chasm,
despair so thick we could palpate the edges
stretching out between us.*

*In honoring that despair, I lifted my hand
in front of our faces, my daughter's and mine,
placing its shape forever in my mind.*

*And she stood there, looking for me to interrupt
this daze, to remember where I was.*

*Standing now before the clerk at the drugstore
who was waiting for me to hand over the money
and purchase these goods—aspirin, dental floss,
and a blood-red collar for a dog who waited
quietly at home far away.*

Trauma was making headlines daily now. People were learning about the symptoms of post-traumatic stress disorder firsthand—survivors, family members who sat by their phones all day, small children who watched on television, rescue workers, New Yorkers who breathed in the fumes and debris for weeks afterward. This illness was going to claim many who did not die.

While researching PTSD, I learned that an elevated sympathetic nervous system caused hyperarousal, which also caused chronic inflammation and altered immune response. Patients with PTSD have increased comorbid depression, anxiety, insomnia, substance abuse, and cancer from altered immune systems. But I did not connect the trauma from 9/11 to the trauma I experienced from listening to patients.

Researchers have discovered that creating a written or verbal account of the trauma is a critical component of healing. Surely one thousand songs met that criteria, but I didn't know what else I needed to do. So I kept on—researching, writing, painting, and working, seeking a solution to a puzzle that was poorly defined.

After reflecting on my years of trauma work, I realized that my sensitivity and intuitiveness had made me susceptible to sustaining post-traumatic stress disorder. Growing up in a family that used physical punishment to shame and control created vulnerability. I thought about Mel, my patients, and myself in light of these findings. Initially, I did not realize how much I had in common with them. But now I began to understand how my reaction to their stories was affecting me. The survival mechanism of walling off the emotions I felt when trauma stories were told had allowed me to walk away seemingly unscathed, and my neutral reactions encouraged patients to trust and continue to tell.

However, the price I paid by compartmentalizing my feelings and blaming God was high.

NORTH CAROLINA

Here's to the land of the long leaf pine,
The summer land where the sun doth shine,
Where the weak grow strong
and the strong grow great.
Here's to "Down Home," the Old North State!
—Leonora Monteiro Martin

TAKING A BREAK FROM THE CLOUDY, dark winters of New Hampshire had been on my agenda for years and seemed imminently possible, as both boys were heading to boarding school in the fall. Alex and I put our heads together and decided that Gray and I could live at the beach for a year. He agreed to fly back and forth between his southern and northern clients, spending as much time in North Carolina as possible. So when we packed for the beach that summer, Gray and I added a few sweaters to the suitcases, leaving our ski coats behind.

I said goodbye to my colleagues at Mental Health Connections after I got a job at a free-standing VA clinic in North Carolina—a new facility that needed a psychiatrist to manage medications for local vets. Seeing men is unusual, because although the need for psychotherapy is gender-blind, men are less likely to seek help.

"This will be stimulating and fun," I said to Alex. "In my years of psychiatric work, I've probably only seen about half a dozen men."

It was interesting, but it wasn't fun. My average patient was a middle-aged veteran exposed to Agent Orange and diagnosed with depression, diabetes, hepatitis, and skin disorders. Multiple medications were prescribed to treat each physical illness, and then they saw me for anti-depressants, anti-anxiety medication, and sleeping pills. I spent much of my time weaning and discontinuing addictive sedative hypnotics and opioids. Sometimes I would spend months getting a patient off their pain pills, only to have them drive three hours to the university emergency room, where the prescription was renewed. Instead of reading my note, the doctor on-call would simply restart the pain med at the dose requested by the patient. If the doctor had accessed the electronic medical record, he would have seen that the taper and discontinuation order were at the veteran's request—how hard we had worked to accomplish that!

Patients came for medication management, but they also brought trauma stories. One older veteran brought war photographs stored for fifty years in a shoe box. Pulling the pictures out one at a time, he named the dead bodies, decapitated heads stuck on stakes, and talked about how they hadn't looked at them in years.

"Dr. Burns, I never took this box out from under my bed before. But now that you're here, I want to show you. I want someone to know. These pictures tell my story of World War II. After the war, I couldn't concentrate or work. I still have nightmares."

Many of the older veterans had never been diagnosed with post-traumatic stress disorder. It was an easy diagnosis to make. Getting the disability was more difficult.

The art of ushering someone in as someone else shuffled out within the twenty minutes allotted was lost on me. And that twenty minutes included the time necessary for writing the patient note and reading the history of the next patient. Veterans often left feeling unsatisfied; their needs were not met. It was frustrating for both of us. Lots of the men asked for Viagra. Here I was seeing male adults and still talking about sex.

"I can't have it. That Agent Orange messed me up, Dr. Burns. Between that, the anti-depressant, and the diabetes, I have to have Viagra. Come on, I know you can write for it."

It was a loud and daily chant.

Of course I could write for Viagra, but I didn't. The nurse practitioner and I had an agreement: she prescribed Viagra so the blood pressure and cardiac side effects in this high-risk population could be monitored in their physical health record. I prescribed psychotropic drugs.

Late one Thursday, a veteran prepared to leave my office. "I give you less than a year, Dr. Burns."

"Why would you say that?"

"The good ones never stay." He walked out of the office.

I thought he was wrong. Time would prove him right.

One of my patients at the VA was being investigated for sexually abusing his son and had pleaded not guilty. I was not involved in the trial and had never met his son, but was treating the veteran for depression, insomnia, and anxiety. He also dissociated and explained that he couldn't feel—afraid that if he felt joy, sadness would consume him and he'd never recover. He chose the void instead. He told me of a time when he stood on the beach and it started to rain.

"Dr. Burns, I could see dark clouds threatening and the rain pouring. I could see drops hitting my hand, but I couldn't feel anything. Nothing. The only way I knew it was raining was to see it. It was strange at first, but now I'm getting used to it. It's the numbness I want to get away from, the nothingness that drives me to think of suicide."

After increasing his anti-depressant, I called a few days later to see how he was, knowing medicine would never be enough.

There were so many patients with trauma, and too few resources to make a difference. It was overwhelming, especially to an intuitive healer. So about thirteen months after I started working at the VA clinic, my mental health started deteriorating again.

MENOPAUSE

I waited and waited and waited for God.
At last he looked; finally he listened.
He lifted me out of the ditch,
pulled me from deep mud.
He stood me up on a solid rock
to make sure I wouldn't slip.
He taught me how to sing the latest God-song,
a praise-song to our God.

—Psalm 40

AND THEN ALONG CAME MENOPAUSE. Living up north disrupted my circadian rhythms, causing winter blues. Secondary trauma led to elevated cortisol and noradrenaline. And menopause created severe insomnia. I had experienced moderate difficulty sleeping for years, but with menopause, I stopped sleeping completely. I went two months without sleeping through the night.

Not realizing that my insomnia was caused by a hyperaroused nervous system, I kept working and exercising. Over-the-counter sleep aids that had worked well through the years were completely ineffective. When I lay down to sleep at night, I felt as if I were plugged into an electrical socket. I was buzzing, no matter how tired I was. Although I had been in supervision throughout my career, now I needed a psychiatrist.

Since I didn't have one, I asked my family doctor, Dr. Brown, for sleeping pills.

"Sleeping pills, Julia?" he said. "Are you stressed?"

"My God, Bill, are you kidding? I work with veterans four days a week and have a private practice one day a week. I take care of my daughter. Alex comes when he can, of course. But yes, I'm stressed." I gave him the only answer I knew.

I wish I could have said, *"Yes, I have a stress disorder from listening to trauma. I'm so jumpy I can't sleep at night. I'm afraid if I don't listen or listen just right or miss something or prescribe the wrong medicine, someone will get hurt. How do I find the pill that makes bad people go away?"*

But not knowing then what I know now, I just kept working and living and loving—getting somewhat better, but not completely well. When menopause hit and I didn't sleep, finally I broke.

I tried calling other providers: "I can't sleep. I stopped menstruating in August and I haven't slept since then. It's October. I need something for sleep."

"Have you tried melatonin?" one asked.

Another said, "How about diphenhydramine or warm milk?"

"I've been using Benadryl and melatonin for years," I said. "Probably ten. I mean, I am not sleeping at all."

"Julia, that's not possible," my nurse practitioner said. "You have to have slept some over the past weeks. After three nights without sleep, you will get paranoid." She refused to prescribe a sleep medication.

Well, it was as if she had made a prophetic announcement, because one week later, paranoia hit. I had gone so long without sleep that my hypervigilant being slipped into psychosis. A place my patients had so often inhabited now claimed me. The good part about having a nervous breakdown is that when you've finally fallen completely into the abyss, you think everyone else is crazy. Then it becomes their problem.

Of course, my first choice would have been to have doctors who did their job by writing me a prescription for sleeping pills to keep my brain from breaking. But my second choice, if it had to happen, was for it to have been just the way it was.

The hand of God was all over us that weekend. Momma was visiting, and my oldest son, Jack, now a freshman in college, was home. Increasingly anxious as the insomnia continued, I was vigilant about my mental deterioration. That Friday, Gray invited her soccer team over for a pizza party, a celebration of the season's victorious end. Momma could help with games and chaperoning, but her limited mobility made it difficult for her to help serve pizza and ice cream. I asked our best friends, Susan and Hugh, to join us, as I felt off-balance and wanted to make sure all went well. Susan and Hugh stayed until the last guest headed home.

That weekend, on the beach, airplanes flew overhead, advertising the latest sunscreen, but they were also watching me. Going to bed that night, I prayed that I would finally sleep. I was exhausted and slightly aware that I was losing my reason. But only slightly—it was too late for me to be my own psychiatrist. I barely closed my eyes.

Sunday morning, while singing in the choir, my fears increased. After our anthem, I was so nervous I picked up my purse, intending to leave the choir loft. Anyone in the congregation could see something was wrong, but nobody knew just how awful it was. No one realized that I saw visions of children being sacrificed on the altar, blood spilling from their suspended bodies. I was sure that it wasn't real—it was more like I *knew* it was happening than actually seeing it. Certain that nobody else saw those sacrifices, I organized myself and sat back down. I didn't tell because I didn't want anyone to think I was mentally ill.

After church, we went out to lunch and things settled down for a while. But later that afternoon, the strange thoughts started again. I called the number off the back of a duct tape roll and told the company that I knew they were following us and they had better not hurt my children. Then I started playing the drums, except there wasn't a drum set. I believe that is when my son decided to call our friends Susan and Hugh, who came and took me to the hospital for an evaluation. And this is where my memory short circuits. The rest of the story about my mad descent comes from my family's account and pieces I've retrieved.

Of course, the doctors in the emergency room thought I was using drugs. The first thing they did was a drug screen, which came back negative. I was sane enough to tell them that, but nobody was listening to me by then.

It was drugs, in a way: after weeks of not sleeping, the release of neurotransmitters and cortisol created a potent drug causing paranoia.

Once they realized I wasn't a druggie, the action picked up. A nurse specialist on-call for psychiatric emergencies did a mental status exam, which I failed miserably, except for orientation. I never lost track of day, date, time, or place. But by then, I was content to tell anyone who asked about the slaughter of our children: "Their blood is all around, and the FBI is using surveillance to keep me quiet."

Eventually, they decided to hospitalize me. If I hadn't been so out of it, I could have told them to give me a sleeping pill and I would be fine. But I *was* out of it and couldn't boss anyone around. The good news is that when your mental status deteriorates over a period of a few days, you can get well just that fast. Jack called Alex, who was at a football game in New York. He drove through the night. After rushing through the hospital parking lot, he pushed past locked doors, barreling into the psychiatric unit after hours.

"They are trying to give me a pill. I think they are poisoning me. Should I take it?"

"Julia, take it," he said. "Do what they say. They are trying to help you."

And that was it. I took my pill and slept for hours.

When I woke up, I said, "I want to go home."

They said, "You haven't been to group therapy or swimming."

As a psychiatrist, I knew they meant it, so I went to group and cut out a Venn diagram and placed my stresses on it. This facilitated a discussion of what I would do when trouble hit. It was completely worthless to me except to facilitate my discharge from the psych unit. Then I went swimming and swam length after length of the pool. (Jack had packed my bathing suit. I'll never know how he knew, but there it was, lying in my suitcase when I needed it.)

When the other patients started getting out of the pool, I got out, too.

Then again I said, "I want to go home."

They said, "OK, let's schedule a follow-up appointment." We arranged that, and I left. As a patient, I got to experience the psychiatric hospital from a different perspective—a view I hope to never see again. Now this, my mental breakdown, is one song I did not want to sing. I was deeply ashamed. When your ankle breaks, you know you'll get casseroles and compassion. But like most psychiatric patients, when my brain broke, I wanted to obfuscate and hide.

The admitting resident told me, "I was so afraid to do your admission, Dr. Burns. I was terrified I would do something wrong and you would notice."

It was amazing how perceptions can differ dramatically. She was admitting a psychotic patient, but in her mind I was a psychiatrist—pretty far from the truth, that night.

"You needn't have worried. I wasn't noticing anything except the FBI surveillance."

"Even crazy, I intimidate people," I told Alex, and repeated the story.

We both laughed.

THE SOUND

> *The fall of dropping water wears away the Stone.*
> —Lucretius

ON THE DAY OF MY DISCHARGE, I sat in my dining room, looking out at my Sunfish sailboat bobbing in the Bogue Sound, yearning for something lost.

> *November's rawness sat inside me*
> *as I reminisced from afar the sunfish sail dance*
> *we had all summer.*
>
> *This boat is moored now between two docks,*
> *yet tomorrow we will haul her out,*
> *scrape sea life off her bottom,*
> *winter her down.*
>
> *But for this one leftover moment,*
> *she will laugh at the chilling air,*
> *jog up and down in the waves,*
> *slapping the sound with a musical swagger.*
>
> *They could bed this way forever*
> *if only we would let them be.*

Putting the pieces together after my hospitalization proved more difficult—the swagger, however musical, was not sustainable. I was admitted over Veteran's Day weekend and never missed a day in my private practice. I kept working one day a week with outpatients after giving up the VA position. They kept calling, but I said no. This time, I was paying attention, not ignoring the breakdown or the insomnia. I was still not sleeping, and the medicine they prescribed made me feel like a mechanical doll: I was stiff, couldn't eat, and felt numb. It's one thing to diagnose the side effects of psychotropic medications and prescribe medicines to counteract them. It's quite another to have those side effects.

The first months after my discharge were strange, and I struggled. I still was not diagnosed correctly, and although I lost thirty pounds, my psychiatrist never weighed me. I kept telling him about the loss of appetite, numbness, and agitation, but he refused to change medicine. He was kind and capable, but deaf to my complaints. It was frustrating to continually have doctors who refused to listen, first accelerating the breakdown, and now treating it incorrectly. I felt invisible, but was too off-balance to advocate for myself.

Everyone commented on how odd I looked.

"Wow, Julia, you look awful. What's wrong? Are you OK?"

"I'm fine. How're you?"

No one believed my deflections. Maybe I should I have said, *"I went crazy after menopause because I didn't sleep for weeks, and now I'm afraid to stop this medicine, terrified it will happen again if I do. I'd rather walk around looking like a zombie. How are you?"*

There never seems to be a good way to talk about mental instability. It's not easy to say, *"My brain broke, and my medicine is hurting me."* The stigma around mental illness is a large part of what makes treatment and recovery so complex.

Finally, switching doctors allowed me to get on a different medicine. In less than two weeks, my life kaleidoscoped into a coherent whole. I moved freely, ate, and gained weight. I also found gratitude and a sense of humor. Only a few of my closest friends knew about my illness. None of them ever mentioned it, except one.

"Julia, you look good. Are you making it or faking it?" she said, one day, when we were walking.

"A bit of both, I guess."

The toil all this took on my family was immeasurable. I played the starring role, and even I cannot comprehend it. My husband—who stood by, watching me go mad, and waiting while I put myself back together—showed enormous patience and love. The children did, too, especially Gray, who was still living at home. I asked their forgiveness for the pain this insanity created for our family. I have forgiven myself, my providers, and God for what happened, as my family has forgiven me. Gray said:

> Mom, I know you don't tell people about your breakdown, but whenever I tell my friends, they say, 'Oh, that happened in our family, too.'
>
> I think everyone knows someone who had a nervous breakdown. It seems normal, at least with my crowd."
>
> Gray urged me not to worry "You are the best mom ever. Remember when I had big tantrums, or when one of us spilled milk and you couldn't clean it up. You were laughing so hard? Remember, Mom? There was always joy.

Memories of their childhood came rushing back, and I couldn't help but compare it to mine. In contrast to my children, I grew up afraid, striving to be perfect, attempting to win Momma's approval to avoid beatings. I've worked hard to forgive the spankings and remember the deep love in our home. Many of the lessons I taught my children, I learned from Momma and Daddy. Both were favored grandparents and loved my children, rarely missing a violin concert, graduation, or birthday, even though they were seven hundred miles away.

I was determined that physical punishment would never be used on my children, and was glad that I had avoided the mistakes my parents made raising me. And I was thankful that I had maintained the good from my childhood.

Though frightening, my descent into madness yielded great dividends. Believing my female menopausal patients' concerns about insomnia was one. Certainly, asking two providers for sleep medication and not getting any relief made me determined to listen to my patients and act. They get immediate attention if they stop sleeping. When anyone mentions insomnia, I educate them regarding sleep hygiene, relaxation, and meditation exercises. I ask them to use lavender sleep cream, Benadryl or melatonin, and essential oil diffusion. If this doesn't work, I prescribe a sleeping pill.

Lesson learned: never leave insomnia untreated. As my nurse practitioner noted, if you don't sleep, you will get paranoid.

Acceptance in full surrender to Christ, and refusing to blame others, was the key to regaining my peace and sanity.

"If you fight reality, refusing to accept it, you will lose, and possibly go mad," a therapist told me, explaining the root cause of my despair and paranoia.

"Dr. Burns, how are you today?" Patient's start their session this way, attempting to avoid their own problems for a few minutes.

"Well, we all have lives, but we're not here to talk about mine. I couldn't charge for that."

We laugh together.

Yes, we all do have lives. And sometimes our lives make us ill. Then it's up to us to make them better.

Although I worked hard to restore my life, it wasn't until years after the hospitalization that I began to understand the phenomenon of secondary PTSD, that I had it and needed treatment.

NO, NOT ME

In order to change, people need to become aware of their sensations and the way that their bodies interact with the world around them. Physical self-awareness is the first step in releasing the tyranny of the past.

—Bessel van der Kolk

FORTUNATELY, IN THE MEDICAL COMMUNITY, as elsewhere, eyes are opening to recognize and name abuse and trauma. As the world cries out for trauma-sensitive care, many are being healed. Memorize the statistic that one in four girls and one in six boys are sexually abused, so the next time someone is rude to you, understanding will come. Hold these numbers in your head and your heart, because it is likely the person annoying you has spent a lifetime of being yelled at or worse. Much worse.

My experiences with the abused informs me that the estimate of one in four girls and one in ten boys is low. Twenty years ago, I began to experiment by asking friends and family if they had been sexually abused.

Many said, "Maybe. I guess so."

Then I asked, "How do you answer that question when asked on a routine questionnaire?"

"No," they reply, surprised at the question.

"I don't think they mean what happened to me," I would hear, "That was showering with my basketball coach. Well, sometimes he did feel me up on the way home from practice, but he was a family friend and my parents trusted him."

Or, "I only made out with my youth director. He was married and lots older, I guess, but we never had intercourse. His wife was always upstairs."

"My father didn't actually abuse us, Dr. Burns. He just made us take off our clothes, then made movies of us dancing naked. But that's not abuse, is it?"

"My Boy Scout leader slept with me in my sleeping bag. He made our troop shower together naked on overnights. But he was the best Scout leader. We biked all over the country."

"My brother and I had sex, but he said we were practicing for marriage and that it didn't count."

"My teacher kept me in for recess if I forgot my homework or talked too much. She fondled me, but that's not really sexual abuse, is it? It's not like we took our clothes off. I remember liking the way it felt and hating it, too. So confusing. I wonder if that's why I'm promiscuous? I don't have boundaries when it comes to relationships, and I can't be faithful. Do you think it's related?"

"The priest masturbated me after buying me an ice cream cone. It melted all down my hands. I never wanted ice cream again after that. He made me eat it. I had no one to tell, Dr. Burns. He was not just my priest, he was my boy scout chaplain, my school chaplain, the chaplain of the fire and police department. On Sundays, he came for lunch and sat beside me, touching me under the table. Who could I tell?"

Here is the truth: rarely in my years of psychiatry has a patient—child or adult—walked into my office and asked for treatment for abuse, physical or sexual. Typically, they seek help for anxiety or depression, and only after months or years in therapy do they remember an incident with an abuser and gain knowledge about how their symptoms relate to trauma.

I once had a patient named Will whose boy scout leader and baseball coach was convicted of distributing child pornography and molesting children. He was sentenced to twenty years in prison. Despite spending years with this man, Will continually refused to consider the possibility that he had been abused. Instead, he was outraged and defended him. Many signs of sexual trauma, including promiscuity and addictions, were present. His life was plagued by volatile, dramatic, and broken relationships, yet Will's denial condemned him to a life controlled by his abuser, even after he was jailed.

My last day working with traumatized children ended with a little girl, Norma, aged eight, who started her appointment by recanting an allegation.

"Dr. Burns, I only told Mom I was having oral sex with Dad to get attention."

She got much attention, but not the kind she needed. Acting as a witness without any power to change, I could stay no longer, and resigned for the last time, reminding Norma that in case her Daddy asked her for oral sex again, she should tell someone besides her mother.

"How about your teacher?" I said.

WHAT HAPPENED TO ME?

> *You groped your way through that murk once,*
> *but no longer. You're out in the open now.*
> *The bright light of Christ makes your way plain.*
> *So no more stumbling around. Get on with it!*
> *The good, the right, the true—these are the*
> *actions appropriate for daylight hours. Figure out*
> *what will please Christ and then do it.*
> —Ephesians 5

ONE LAST STORY MAY HELP COMPLETE THE PUZZLE of my life and answer the question as to why I became a trauma specialist. Several years ago, I was at a family reunion and we were talking about work and children, and the subject of childhood trauma surfaced. Several of my relatives recounted their own sexual molestations.

"When I was little, an older relative sexually abused me. Ellen was twelve and I was six when she molested me. The abuse was constant, since we lived close by."

I was shocked but not surprised, having run towards and away from this knowledge as it molded my life. The room started swimming, and my hearing got wonky. I wanted everyone to slow down, or stop talking, or keep talking forever. Here was the explanation for which I had been searching.

I said nothing.

"Don't you remember the barn?" someone asked me. "Playing the milking game?"

"I don't remember. Tell me, was I there?" I asked several times if I had been there, if anyone had ever seen me playing the milking game, and what exactly was the milking game, but no one wanted to talk further.

That door had closed, and it wasn't going to open again. We talked in generalities after that.

I asked them why they never told anyone, and the answer was, "Julia, who would we have told? Who would have listened?"

And knowing this truth so well, I only nodded.

I could think of little else, and wanted more—more information, more confirmation, and especially more evidence about my involvement.

"Was I there?" I asked others. "Did I see or experience anything?"

"Be grateful, Julia, that you don't remember. God has graced you with that."

But it didn't feel like grace. It felt like a dead end, and the red bird wasn't singing her song. Of course, I had wondered if I had ever experienced childhood trauma, my body remembering what my mind had shut away—emotions so powerful and experiences so damaging that conscious memory was suppressed. But knowing is different from wondering, and now I had a testimony that there were sexual boundary violations in my family. It felt unfair that God had favored me with the gift of seeing, hearing, and feeling the abuse stories of others, yet I was drawing a blank on my own. It was time to get back into therapy. I wanted to be hypnotized, given medicine to help me remember. I'd do anything to learn the truth.

Slowly, I have come to believe that since listening to, believing, and protecting children has defined me, it was likely my childhood narrative also. Perhaps as a young child, I heard or saw sexual activity that frightened me. I may have tried to get help, but the adults failed to listen and protect. My body then locked tight these secrets long before I worked as a psychiatrist, creating the backdrop for my belief that patients were telling the truth—my listening informed by what I had heard or seen. Other days, I'm not sure.

Sexual trauma caused deep ancestral wounds in my family that I was born to redeem each time I diagnosed and treated a child. I believe my relatives were looking down, applauding. I pray that the listening and believing over thirty years has healed this generational brokenness in some small but substantial manner.

"What if I had wanted to be a ballerina?" I asked my therapist, perhaps hoping that I could be emancipated from this listening, this knowing, this understanding about so many, and now of myself.

She only shook her head.

It may not be predestination, but it's pretty close. I have come to accept it.

GENERATIONAL PATTERNS

Harm and heartache are an inevitable part of the human experience, but all too often we lack the tools to care for our wounds well, and the trauma leaves a lasting mark on our body, mind, and soul.

—Dan Allender
Healing the Wounded Heart

"Hey, Alex, they are finally starting to study secondary PTSD," I said, one night, as we were reading after supper.

Researchers had recently described symptoms of hyperarousal, hypervigilance, exaggerated startle, and emotional numbing as "normal responses for therapists." As the autonomic nervous system goes into overdrive, they explained, it impairs health. Under chronic stress, the sympathetic nervous system produces adrenaline and noradrenaline. This alters the genetic code, leading to PTSD, impaired immune response, and a number of physical diseases.

Scientists were finally delineating a syndrome I knew too well. My inbox filled with resources for treating vicarious PTSD: Breathing exercises were recommended to decrease the effects of cortisol, lessening the damage of the fight-or-flight reaction. Conferences reviewing the effects of secondary PTSD and its treatment were burgeoning. Polyvagal theory delineating ventral vagal (relaxed), sympathetic (fight or flight) and dorsal vagal (numb, dissociated) was being used to treat flashbacks, discern triggers, and map neurological responses so moving up and down the ladder of neurological arousal could be a learned behavior and not a reflex.

"At last, someone is studying trauma in therapists and attempting to treat it," I said.

"Julia, I guess so. I don't really understand that medical mumbo jumbo, but I can see how listening to trauma stories would set you up for PTSD. Makes a lot of sense."

At long last, professors are educating medical students on how to care for themselves, acknowledging that vicarious traumatization occurs in 50 percent of medical students during a psychiatry rotation. Students exhibit avoidance of social activities, flashbacks, nightmares, memory deficits, and feelings of horror and shame. They experience God as uncaring, and exhibit irritability, hyper-vigilance, paranoia, anxiety, and mood swings. Medical student psychiatry rotations last six weeks. Mine has lasted years.

I'm glad scientists are studying secondary PTSD and helping therapists ameliorate the effects of stress, but I doubt if foreknowledge would have made a major difference in my case. It would be like saying, *If you know how car accidents cause whiplash and you get rear ended, your neck will not hurt.*

Sometimes parents are just not able to be *good enough* because of their own childhood wounds. Usually, parents do not want to abuse their children. However, changing generational patterns requires intention and assistance. Research shows that abused, neglected, and poorly attached children grow up to be anxious, fearful, and much less able to assess danger. These traits lead to more traumatization. High-risk families are easily identified so programs in labor and delivery can offer support. Questionnaires gauge poverty, drug or alcohol addiction, family structure (single head of household is a risk factor), history of mental illness, and abuse histories. Two or more positive responses allows eligibility. The best programs are voluntary, and the majority of people agree to participate. Families are shown how to play with their children, change diapers, soothe infants when they cry, and make and show up for medical appointments. Families that enroll in the preventative program bring their rates of abuse from 16–24 percent to less than 1 percent.[9]

When caregivers fail to soothe and settle their infants, insecure attachment occurs, which is the most common attachment style seen in my trauma patients. These children are easily frightened, unable to distinguish between a happy or angry expression, and unable to engage with others. Insecure attachments breed fear. Soothing babies instead of agitating them allows infants to connect with caregivers, increasing their chance for a secure bond. When caregivers are unresponsive, the child has to deal with anxiety on their own. Either they become agitated and upset, or passive and withdrawn.

So you see, support is needed in infancy. Waiting to intervene when children are school age is often too late. Without instruction on interactive play, we can predict that infants will experience poor attachment, becoming disruptive and aggressive. This will increase the likelihood that they will be abused. The abuse often goes undocumented until the child starts school.

We possess the tools capable of predicting and preventing abuse. Yet we continue to fall short and fail future generations—building prisons, despite evidence that they are not effective in changing behavior. Refusing to nurture and treat marginalized, traumatized families is an acting out of our culture's unresolved hurts as we turn a blind eye to their needs. We are all wounded people searching for ways to heal.

Knowledge that poor parenting begets more poor parenting, which creates poorly attached humans, which leads to anxiety, depression, and abuse, is a simple theory, but it places much responsibility on us. The solutions are within reach, yet we fail to use them to break the cycle. Instead, we judge and punish, our fear alienating us from each other and from solutions that would create radical advancements in our ability to protect and care for each other.

COMPLEX TRAUMA

The first principle of recovery is empowerment of the survivor. She must be the author and arbiter of her own recovery. Others may offer advice, support, assistance, affection, and care, but not cure.

—Judith Herman

THE NATIONAL CHILD TRAUMATIC STRESS NETWORK states that complex trauma describes both children's exposure to multiple traumatic events—often of an invasive, interpersonal nature—and the wide-ranging, long-term effects of this exposure. These events are severe and pervasive, and include abuse or profound neglect. They usually occur early in life and can disrupt many aspects of the child's development and the formation of a sense of self. Many treatment modalities, residential and outpatient centers for complex trauma victims, focus on wraparound programs that improve function and decrease symptoms.[10]

But what are best practices for reducing abuse, for treating it after it happens? Identifying families who need support by treating and eliminating addictions and mentoring good parenting is often the first step. If we now know that in order for trauma survivors to reclaim their lives they must remember and process how their abusive experiences shaped them, how do we create opportunities for this to happen? Individual and group therapy, medications, energy therapy, and somatic therapy are available treatments. However, after decades of caring for patients, I have come to realize that healing doesn't lie in words alone, and is rarely found in a bottle of pills. In order to stop this epidemic, caregivers and community leaders have to educate themselves and become aware of risk factors, creating grass roots prevention programs.

Not long ago, while conducting a Christ-centered conversation about sexual violence at a church, the pastor said, "I'm sorry I couldn't promote your speech with the congregation. We just had a sexual abuse scandal with the boy scouts in the church, and I couldn't make the announcement. It was too painful."

I wondered if I had heard her correctly. Was there any way her words could be translated into something coherent or logical? But there was no justification for her position, and my experience affirms that secrets and denial are what perpetrators rely on and manipulate so expertly.

Instinctively, we wall off pain, creating an exile, because re-experiencing and remembering darkness takes courage. As we hide behind a façade of untruths, wounds are exacerbated, whether we are victims, perpetrators, or silent observers. Healing requires intentional remembering, lamenting, forgiveness, and reconciliation, for ourselves and others. Although the timing must be determined by the survivor, when we choose to skip any of these steps, we too often re-create abuse in our lives and in our loved one's lives, despite vowing that this is the last thing we want.

The anguish serial molester Dr. Larry Nassar experienced when faced with the testimonies of his victims supports that he was possibly dissociating when he abused his patients. He demonstrated this in the courtroom during the gymnasts' testimonies by asking the judge to excuse him because he was *too distressed* and could not tolerate more. It was as if he were experiencing the women's *suffering* for the first time.

Treating perpetrators as victims of childhood trauma honors human life. Further violation of their humanity, which repeats the shame and condemnation of their childhood, combined with imprisonment, rarely interrupts the cycle. A hurtful childhood filled with manipulation and judgement takes much therapy and hard work to overcome. A childhood of physical and sexual abuse takes even more hard work, and if healing is not purposeful, then patterns may be repeated.

As perpetrators and victims take responsibility for their lives and the direction in which they want to grow, critical changes will take place in individuals and in cultural norms. As perpetrators listen to victims' stories of abuse, they must apologize for the hurt they've caused. As victims forgive at their own pace, they can disentangle themselves from their abusers. The questions must be asked: Who am I besides perpetrator? Who am I besides victim?

When I was a young doctor, I heard a judge tell a two-year-old that if she hadn't shaken her tushy at her grandfather, he would not have raped her—*not guilty*. Incredulous at this callous and ridiculous theory, I thought if I could stand in for that judge, I would send all perpetrators to jail. That will show them, I thought. That will take care of the problem.

However, in my last stint in the prison system, I interviewed and treated many perpetrators, and now realize how naive that thinking was, because the jails are full of perpetrators.

"Dr. Burns, if they look like white-collar workers and say they are in for embezzlement, you can be pretty sure they are child molesters."

Many prisoners fit that description, yet each night we watch the news as another teen with a history of trauma shoots his classmates, or an infant is found brutally murdered by an abused mother. We watch courtroom scenes as a female teacher is sentenced to fifteen years for molesting a young student. Or a famous musician builds a child's fantasyland to lure his victims, and no one asks questions, even the parents, when he sleeps with the children in his bed.

With too few mental health clinics and not nearly enough psychiatrists, physically abused and sexually traumatized children and teens often go untreated. Incarcerating perpetrators, although perhaps necessary, is never going to be sufficient.

HEALING PRAYER

O my soul, bless God. From head to toe, I'll bless his holy name. O my soul, bless God, don't forget a single blessing! He heals your diseases—every one.
—Psalm 103

WHEN I CONSIDER MY CONSTELLATION of characteristics, genetics, and environment, I don't wonder that I had a paranoid episode. I wonder how I made it forty-seven years before it occurred. Fighting reality made me lose my mind. In many ways, I'm glad it did, because it brought me to a place of surrender that I never would have reached without it. A place so peaceful it surpasses all understanding, because it lies outside my humanness and within the depths of my Creator.

Most of my creations originated through Spirit, and I am deeply grateful for the gifts of writing and painting as my pen and paintbrush re-create traumatic narratives. Using all my senses to learn so others know and understand that light can shine and penetrate the blackness that encloses so many. When I paint healing meditations for trauma survivors, their songs are covered in colors. This brings a realness and vibrancy to their stories.

Although art, medication, and psychotherapy partially healed me, in the end, it was God who orchestrated my full recovery. God who came down from heaven and entered my heart, releasing me from my self-imposed burden to create a world free of trauma.

My close relationship with God led to a passion for healing prayer. This enthusiasm was intensified years later when my church's healing prayer team used this treatment modality to fight my cancer. After being diagnosed with systemic, rare and aggressive inflammatory breast cancer, my chance of surviving more than two years was less than 25 percent. I used chemotherapy, surgery, radiation, nutrition, exercise, essential oils, and meditation, and eventually I was healed.

Now, healing prayer, along with traditional psychotherapy, medication, cognitive therapy, and somatic energy techniques, are common in my psychiatric practice. Verbal therapy, which targets the frontal cortex, is limited in its effectiveness, especially when the traumas occurred before language was acquired, or the terror is so great that language is lost. When a patient makes a connection between a symptom (smelling donuts) and a traumatic event (rape) during talk therapy or a somatic energy treatment, we seal the learning and discovery with prayer, asking that light cover the knowledge so donuts can be enjoyed again.

Dissociation, a common defense against chronic trauma, is uncovered, and at each appointment, fuzzy, vague memories are analyzed for specific details, because healing lies in the specificity. Research on the use of virtual reality re-creating war atrocities revealed that the more concrete facts the patient can remember about their trauma, the deeper and more sustaining the symptom reduction.[11] Conscious remembering stops the repetition of dysfunctional behaviors, so no matter how painful the retrieval, the goal to recollect must persist. While praying with and for my patients, I know that God weeps with us and never causes our suffering. But he can aid our remembering, reduce our symptoms, and redeem our traumas—if we ask him.

Recently, a study was conducted with subjects who transcribed their trauma stories and then replayed the trauma in their head multiple ways, as if in a "movie"—first forward, then in black and white, then backwards.[12] Afterwards, their life-threatening events seemed less frightening, and participants' symptoms improved. This improvement was present in follow-up months later.[13]

Another intervention asks patients to bring a "protector" to walk through a specific dark memory. This makes people feel less vulnerable, less alone. I speculate that inviting Christ into a memory changes it, perhaps in a similar manner. Or if they don't believe in Christ or a higher power, then perhaps another "superpower"—an adult from their childhood, who seemed safe and strong—might be able to join them in reliving their trauma memory, creating a sense of separateness and safety.

"Is it possible that darkness is holding you back, exacerbating some symptoms?"

Usually, I hear, "Yes. Please, Dr. Burns, I want to feel better."

"Can we pray about this?"

"Yes, let's pray."

And we pray together, asking love and light to dispel negativity and darkness in the spiritual domain, laying aside fear.

Combining healing prayer with traditional psychotherapy, medication, and energy practices has resulted in dramatic responses in my post-traumatic stress disordered patients. Often, there is a rapid reduction in the following: insomnia, hypervigilance, paranoia, headaches, memory lapses, and emotional isolation. Patients return to work faster and find new enjoyment in routine tasks. Obsessive compulsive thoughts and rituals dissipate.

Regrettably, in past years of listening to patients and taking histories, completing psychiatric evaluations, and prescribing medications, I never worked with an organization that assessed spirituality. Until recently, I never even asked patients if they believed in God and how that influenced their thinking and feeling.

Occasionally, I asked, "What religion are you?"

Recording Methodist or Presbyterian on a form was where it ended. Worship and church communities, youth leaders, ministers, prayers, and God were not listed as resources, and I mourn missing that opportunity.

Presently, about half of my patients want to use all modalities of healing, including spiritual ones.

So I say, "I pray to God regularly for insight, healing, and courage for myself and would be happy to do the same for you. If you don't yet practice prayer, perhaps you would like to try. I believe that God cares and replies in many different ways."

Now, with each new patient evaluation, I ask, "Do you see yourself as a religious or spiritual person? Has your problem affected you spiritually? What was your spiritual background as a child? Are you part of a religious or spiritual community? Have you had experiences of love or the presence of the divine? Would you like to use spiritual or religious resources in your therapy?"

Often, I see patients who have been wounded by religion and its ministers. They find seeking God's guidance difficult, and many sessions are needed before acknowledgement that humans, not God, caused the wound. Sometimes that acknowledgement never comes, and healing is stalled. We need all the might we can muster to create a safer place for children, because sadly, evil exists everywhere, including the church. When abuse is perpetrated deep in the recesses of God's holy temples, it is particularly powerful. Victims become convinced that hatred and fear conquer forgiveness and love. But this is never true, even when the abuse is done in the name of God, in his church.

God does not perpetrate evil, nor does he condone it. Blanket condemnation of the church causes great harm, as corporate worship is one of the most powerful weapons we have against darkness—God loves it when we sing praises. However, darkness does penetrate and attempt to take over churches. Sexual perversions and abuses infiltrating the church seek to destroy it.

After years of wrestling with God, I now believe that trauma survivors hold a special place in his heart. And although

God did create the world and everything in it, he does not condone child abuse, and intercedes in every way possible to counter it. Look at this book as one of those ways.

GENERATIONAL HEALING

Pain travels through family lines until someone is ready to heal it in themselves. By going through the agony of healing, you no longer pass the poison chalice onto the generations that follow. This is incredibly important and sacred work.

—Anonymous

TIME DOES NOT HEAL, IT CONCEALS. Remember how involved I was in the ministry of the church when I was wounded? Remember how no one knew or wanted to know, and how I settled into a temporary façade of "normal"? Unfortunately, churches have been slow to understand the depth of suffering among its members. Church can be just another place we go to pretend.

Passing the peace is a cursory obligation of, *"Hi, I'm fine. And you?"* Members are rarely invited to claim healing or tell their stories. Instead, church is the place where we dress up and continue the pretext of how good God is and how great he has been. There is little discussion on how difficult life is and how God could have allowed such chaos. Yet it is the church's job to gain entry into the world of healing without creating fear.

"The church is not preaching the gospel unless it is engaged in healing work," says Francis McNutt, a spiritual leader and healer.

How and when is the church going to step with authority into its role as healer? When will they proclaim the power of healing prayer as loudly as they ask for money during the offering? Are they ever going to expose church members and leaders when they act as perpetrators or ignorant enablers?

Recently, a generational communion for families was held in my church. After prayer and meditation, worshippers diagrammed their family tree, going back five generations, listing wounds, weaknesses, and strengths. Ministers invited participants to take communion, bring their family diagrams and leave them on the altar. The ministers blessed the family histories and then burned them, effectively burning and releasing hurts and wounds that had caused suffering for decades.

Naming my family's problems—obesity, food addictions, diabetes, high blood pressure, peripheral neuropathy, sexual abuse, pornography, racism, jealousy, sibling rivalry, cancer, resentment, bitterness, lack of forgiveness, pride, addiction, and physical abuse—I diagrammed wounds. I named gifts like service to others, gratitude, cheerfulness, love of Christ, good health, hospitality, intelligence, beauty, creative and musical talent. After heading to the altar for communion, my heart lightened and peace enveloped me as I laid my family tree on the altar. Walking away, I felt connected to my ancestors.

Surely God listens, cares, and wants to restore our lives. But we have to help. This fight against trauma and violence demands our awareness and intention, because without our eyes that see, our ears that hear, and our tongues that report and tell, God is without soldiers in this battle. So here we are together, telling, listening, and changing the world as Christ, the consummate listener and storyteller, cheers us on from his seat at the right hand of God, where he intercedes for us and for all victims. Forever.

As I continue to practice medicine and listen to trauma stories, they no longer wound me, because now I listen not with my ears, but with the heart of Christ. And the blessings of wisdom, compassion, and understanding are bestowed on both patient and doctor by a benevolent Creator who knew about abuse before time began.

Spiritual Catharsis

Standing at the edge of the end of that year,
the year of the angel's garden visitation,
the year of a thousand songs,

Standing at the end of that year of emptying,
I longed for a graduation,
yearned for a celebration commemorating
the death of a doctor, the birth of an artist,
and the life that was yet to come.

The year thousands of songs erupted.
I wanted to empty myself even more,
wanted to make myself small, insignificant,
or maybe wanted to be swallowed
by something larger than me and my prayers.

So I planned a trip to the grandest canyon,
the seventh wonder of the world,
and our family journeyed west to face that abyss.

Let the movement of her river cut me
like it had that rock, six thousand feet deep
and into my soul.

Swallow me and make me whole.

Red clay, black rock, river canyon,
separate my spirit like the water did you.

Allow my entry, then send me downriver
and back home, but not to my death.

Explorers run the river to see where it goes,
to chart its path and to make history.

I wrote one thousand songs to see where I was,
where I was going, to chart my path and maybe to
make a history.

*Navigating my raft
through that muddy red river,
letting the current pull me down,
watching the white water sweep up
and over my beloveds, dipping and swaying
to the tug of the rapid's dance,
feeling the sun and wind burn my face,
sear my heart and swell my soul,
I know that I am like that river,
that I continue to create, because like that rock, I
give way to the acid's burning and cutting,
give way to the sculpting and shaping of my soul.*

*Journeying to the red rock canyon,
I stretched out over that ten-mile expanse,
climbed the falls to bathe red dust off my breasts
—cleanse and release—then rappelled back
down the rocks and away.*

*Standing at the edge, singing with the many
on Easter morning as the sun rose
over her distant walls,
I felt free, not diminished, but part of something
far greater than I could fathom.*

*While holding my daughter's hand in mine, we intoned,
Christ the Lord is Risen today.*

Hallelujah.

Stand at the edge of the abyss.

*Feel the wind and the water. Let the acid cut your
soul, setting you free.*

*Celebrate the end of this year and your
new beginning.*

—Julia W. Burns, MD

ACKNOWLEDGEMENTS

THE AUTHOR WISHES TO ACKNOWLEDGE the following for their help with this book: Ivan, Robert, Katy, Pat, Dawn, Leigh Anne, Meghan, and Wally.

With respect and appreciation to my patients, who taught me all I know about trauma, perseverance, and healing.

With never-ending gratitude to my family for living through these struggles and triumphs and loving me to the end.

And to all readers of these words, who will create transformation with their knowledge.

Connect with Dr. Burns at:
www.juliaburns.org

ENDNOTES

1. Meyers, John E.B. "(PDF) A Short History of Child Protection in America." Accessed April 10, 2020. https://www.researchgate.net/publication/254142517_A_Short_History_of_Child_Protection_in_America.

2. Freedman, Alfred M., Harold I. Kaplan, and Benjamin J. Sadock. Comprehensive Textbook of Psychiatry, II. Baltimore, MD: Williams and Wilkins, 1975.

3. Midgley, Nick. Reading Anna Freud. Routledge, 2013.

4. A., Van der Kolk Bessel. The Body Keeps the Score: Brain, Mind, and Body in the Healing of Trauma. NY, NY: Penguin Books, 2015.

5. Sroufe, L. Alan. The Development of the Person: the Minnesota Study of Risk and Adaption from Birth to Adulthood. New York: Guilford Press, 2009.

6. Sroufe, L. Alan. "Attachment and Development: A Prospective, Longitudinal Study from Birth to Adulthood." Attachment & Human Development 7, no. 4 (2005).

7. "Adverse Childhood Experiences (ACEs)." Accessed October 20, 2016. http://www.cdc.gov/violenceprevention/acestudy.

8. "Funeral Blues by W H Auden." by W H Auden - Famous poems, famous poets. - All Poetry. Accessed April 10, 2020. https://allpoetry.com/Funeral-Blues.

9. Yuenger, James. "Hawaii Reduces Abuse With Early Intervention" chicagotribune.com, September 1, 2018. https://www.chicagotribune.com/news/ct-xpm-1993-07-25-9307250310-story.html.

10. Peterson, Sarah. "Complex Trauma." The National Child Traumatic Stress Network, May 25, 2018. https://www.nctsn.org/what-is-child-trauma/trauma-types/complex-trauma.

11. Efficacy of Virtual Reality Exposure Therapy in the Treatment of PTSD: A Systematic Review. Raquel Gonçalves, Ana Lúcia Pedrozo, Evandro Silva Freire Coutinho, Ivan Figueira, and Paula Ventura (PLoS One. 2012; 7(12): e48469.) Published online 2012 Dec 27. doi: 10.1371/journal.pone.0048469. PMCID: PMC3531396. PMID: 23300515.

12. Bandler, R. (2019, July 03). NLP Technique: NLP Fast Phobia Cure. Retrieved July 02, 2020, from https://www.nlp-techniques.org/what-is-nlp/fast-phobia-cure.

13. Bellini, Paul and Michael Roy. "RECONsolidation of Traumatic Memories to ResOLve Post Traumatic Stress Disorder (RECONTROLPTSD) - Full Text View," 2019. https://clinicaltrials.gov/ct2/show/NCT03827057.

www.ingramcontent.com/pod-product-compliance
Lightning Source LLC
Chambersburg PA
CBHW032150080426
42735CB00008B/654